HERMENEUTIC
PHENOMENOLOGICAL
RESEARCH

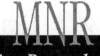

Methods in Nursing Research

SERIES EDITOR
Pamela Brink, R.N., Ph.D.

The purpose of the **Research Methods in Nursing** series is to provide basic references to designs, methods, and sampling procedures not readily available in other formats. Each book is designed to be a complete reference to any single topic.

Books in This Series . . .

Ethnography in Nursing Research
Janice M. Roper
Jill Shapira

Hermeneutic Phenomenological Research
Marlene Z. Cohen
David L. Kahn
Richard H. Steeves

HERMENEUTIC PHENOMENOLOGICAL RESEARCH

A Practical Guide for
Nurse Researchers

Marlene Zichi Cohen
David L. Kahn
Richard H. Steeves

MNR
Methods in Nursing Research

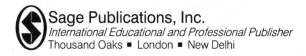

Sage Publications, Inc.
International Educational and Professional Publisher
Thousand Oaks ▪ London ▪ New Delhi

For information:

Sage Publications, Inc.
2455 Teller Road
Thousand Oaks, California 91320
E-mail: order@sagepub.com

Sage Publications Ltd.
6 Bonhill Street
London EC2A 4PU
United Kingdom

Sage Publications India Pvt. Ltd.
M-32 Market
Greater Kailash I
New Delhi 110 048 India

Printed in the United States of America

Library of Congress Cataloging-in-Publication Data

Cohen, Marlene Zichi.
  Hermeneutic phenomenological research: A practical guide for nurse researchers / by Markene Zichi Cohen, David L. Kahn, and Richard H. Steeves.
      p. cm. — (Methods in nursing research; v. 2)
  Includes bibliographical references and index.
    ISBN 0-7619-1719-5 (cloth : alk. paper) — ISBN 0-7619-1720-9 (pbk. : alk. paper)
    1. Nursing—Research. 2. Phenomenology. 3. Hermeneutics. 4. Qualitative research. I. Kahn, David L. II. Steeves, Richard H. III. Title. IV. Series.
    RT81.5 .C63 2000
    610.73'07'2—dc21   00-009007

This book is printed on acid-free paper.

00   01   02   03   04   05   06   7   6   5   4   3   2   1

Acquiring Editor:	Margaret H. Seawell
Editorial Assistant:	Sandra Krumholz
Production Editor:	Diane S. Foster
Editorial Assistant:	Cindy Bear
Typesetter:	Barbara Burkholder
Cover Designer:	Michelle Lee

CONTENTS

SERIES EDITOR'S FOREWORD

Nursing science has had a relatively short history when compared to the other professions. Much of its scientific method has been borrowed from other disciplines and other schools of thought. As a result, nursing has had to adapt research methodologies developed for and by other disciplines to suit nursing problems. Early in nursing scientific history, therefore, nurses used the experimental design and the sociological method of surveys. Frequently, however, the questions that interest nurses involve what is known as "soft" data or data that are not directly amenable to counting and mathematical manipulation. Instead, nursing often asks questions about people and how they are living with their illness or treatment. To answer those questions, nurses turned to qualitative research methods.

Nursing then wanted to know which qualitative research method is the best one to use. That question, of course, is too simplistic. The question should be which qualitative research method is the best one to answer the question I am asking. Once again, however, nursing borrowed research methodologies from other disciplines, methodologies that had been developed to answer that discipline's questions. To answer nursing questions, the methodologies needed to be adapted. The proliferation of articles on qualitative research methods and the disagreement among researchers as to how to conduct certain types of research have led to the development of this research series.

There are many research methods available to answer nursing research questions. None is intrinsically good or bad. Each has its usefulness and limitations. To do a specific piece of research, however, the researcher needs to be familiar with the particular method and how it can help to answer the question being asked. This series of books is attempting to provide serious researchers with the information they need to select the appropriate research method for a particular project. Because no single method is adequate to answer all questions and because no single researcher is equally good at all methods, these books provide an in-depth resource for serious scholars.

Hermeneutic Phenomenological Research is a guide to the conduct of phenomenological research using the philosophical underpinnings of hermeneutics.

There are many forms of phenomenological research, many different philosophical positions on phenomenology, and many teachers of phenomenological research methods. This text takes one position and describes it in its entirety. The first chapter gives an excellent overview of phenomenological research, its historical antecedents, and its philosophical underpinnings. The authors move from this introduction into the "how to" of doing research using this method. The chapters are in the same logical sequence they would follow in any basic research text. This is a "stand alone" text and can be used by first-time researchers who wish to learn to use this method. The text is also useful as a resource and reference for advanced researchers.

One of the unusual aspects of this book is that the three coauthors have maintained their individuality throughout the book. Each author writes in a different "voice" or style. Yet all authors have agreed to the content and substance of each chapter as it fits the work as a whole.

Marlene Cohen, David Kahn, and Richard Steeves have collaborated on a number of phenomenological studies. They are a research team. They have been well funded both locally and federally for their work. The book uses their own work as examples of the method. Because they are a team, the book naturally exemplifies team research. Hermeneutic phenomenology can be done by single investigators as well as by a team of investigators, as the authors point out. I believe you will find this a fascinating book.

—Pamela J. Brink, RN, PhD
Series Editor

PREFACE

Have you ever read a book and wondered about the process the authors used to create it? We are about to tell you about the process that we used to write this book. You will notice that each chapter has a named author. This book is not quite an edited book. We worked together to outline the contents of the book, that is, the topics of each chapter. We then divided the work of writing each chapter, and each wrote his or her part. When we sent our chapters to each other, it was clear that we each used very different writing styles. We decided not to edit out our differences for two reasons. First, writing and individuality are very important in hermeneutic phenomenological research. (We will describe our method in far more detail throughout this book, especially in Chapter 1.) Second, the students I was working with at the time we wrote the first draft of this book read the draft and said they spent a great deal of time trying to figure out who wrote which part. For both of these reasons, we decided to acknowledge our differences and contributions up front and keep our individual styles. We each contributed to all of the chapters. We each read, critiqued, and helped add content to the chapters we did not write. Also, because we have worked together, some of what we wrote has come from that shared work.

We wrote this book for nurses, both graduate students and practitioners, who have some knowledge and experience with research but who are new to phenomenological research. One of the reviewers of an earlier version of this book suggested it could be used as a text or text supplement for researchers at all levels. We have each conducted a number of studies and, to write the book, we have drawn from our research and from our teaching of research to doctoral students. The chapters stand alone and thus can be read in any order. We have, however, organized them in an order that we thought would most logically lead readers through the process of conducting their first hermeneutic phenomenological research project.

We wrote more about teamwork in this book. I do want to begin by acknowledging that working with this team of authors was, as always, a pleasure. Because we work in different cities, as we each wrote chapters, we e-mailed text to each other. I also want to acknowledge and thank Mrs. Nancy Villarreal for her expert assistance putting these chapters together and resolving formatting problems.

We hope you enjoy reading this as much as we have enjoyed writing it.

Marlene Z. Cohen

This book is dedicated to my mentors, colleagues, students, and informants from whom I have learned so much, and especially to my husband, David M. Cohen, who has made the journey so much more fun.

—Marlene Z. Cohen

This book is dedicated to our teacher and friend, Jeanne Quint Benoliel.

—David L. Kahn
—Richard H. Steeves

1

INTRODUCTION

MARLENE Z. COHEN

This chapter will orient the reader to hermeneutic phenomenological research. When and why the method is useful will be discussed and illustrated with examples from the authors' research. The importance and usefulness of this method for nursing research will be discussed, along with the questions that are most appropriate for this design, that is, questions of the meaning of experience. Because phenomenology is the study of lived experience, this idea will be discussed (Husserl, 1970; Schutz & Luckmann, 1973) and contrasted with other experiences, such as reflected or vicarious experiences. A brief orientation to the philosophy of science, from which phenomenology draws its assumptions, and a historical sketch of phenomenological research will also be presented in this chapter. When, why, and how this method started will be described, along with the major schools of phenomeno-logical philosophy and method. Finally, some orientation to issues of language will be provided. For example, phenomenologists would not likely use the word *subjects*. Several other words that are more likely to be used are interchangeable, such as *informants, participants,* or *patients.*

GETTING STARTED

Beginning is never easy and requires many forms of preparation. I re-cently reread Steinbeck's discussion of preparing for a trip, and perhaps because writing this chapter was on my mind, his discussion sounded much like preparing to begin research. In my case the researcher, for Steinbeck (1986) the traveler,

> must first find in himself [sic] a good and sufficient reason for going. . . . Next he must plan his trip in time and space, choose a direction and a desti-nation. And last he must implement the journey. How to go, what to take, how long to stay. This part of the process is invariable and immortal. I set it down only so that newcomers . . . will not think they invented it. (pp. 3-4)

As he continued to discuss the journey, the parallels with research again struck me.

> An exploration is an entity, different from all other journeys. It has person-ality, temperament, individuality, uniqueness. A journey is a person in it-self; no two are alike. And all plans, safeguards, policing, and coercion are fruitless. . . . We do not take a trip; a trip takes us . . . a journey is like mar-riage. The certain way to be wrong is to think you control it. I feel better now, having said this, although only those who have experienced it will understand it. (p. 4)

Yes, beginning research is like beginning a journey, which is like a marriage. With luck, both are worth the time and trouble, and what re-searchers learn about themselves along the way is often the most impor-tant part of the process. In research, as in marriages, having wonderful partners with whom to share the process is both useful and helpful. These partners will make the journey more fun and a better and richer experience.

So, as you begin your journey, why might you choose to begin with phenomenological research? Of course, the first lesson learned in research classes is that the research design should match the question asked. Phenomenological research is used to answer questions of meaning. This method is most useful when the task at hand is to understand an experience as it is understood by those who are having it. Phenomenological research is an important method with which to begin when studying a new topic, or a topic that has been studied but for which a fresh perspective is needed. We illustrate this text with examples from our programs of research, which include a variety of phenomenological projects.

One example that illustrates these points is the study we conducted to understand better what it is like for women to have surgery for breast cancer (Cohen, Kahn, & Steeves, 1998). We asked women to talk about what having breast cancer was like for them. These interviews were transcribed verbatim to construct texts for analysis. When we analyzed these texts, the journey took us to their experiences of their body. The ways that they talked about their bodies went beyond what is traditionally thought about when *body image* is discussed. This study led us to describe a fresh perspective of body image. Our informants described for us what they experienced and, in doing so, gave us a different perspective of body image than the perspectives previously described in the literature. This was not precisely what we had in mind—we did not set out to study body image—but that was where our informants took us. The journey led us to a place we neither controlled nor predicted.

This example also illustrates that our research was the study of the lived experience of these women. We asked them to describe an experience they had lived, not a vicarious experience or a reflection on their experience. Phenomenology is the study of phenomena, as opposed to noumena, using Kant's distinction (summarized in Roche, 1973). *Noumena* are the things themselves, the physical, unchanging, and concrete things as compared to the *phenomena,* our experience of the things. An example is a desk: The desk itself is the noumenon, and our experience of the desk, the phenomenon, is how we perceive that desk. If there were only phenomena, we would run the risk of bumping into the desk each time we passed it. However, we share the intersubjective experience of its existence. If you sit behind my desk, you see piles of papers arranged so that only I can find what I need. If you enter my study, you see one end of a wooden desk, file cabinets blocking the other end, a computer, and, of course, those piles of papers. From behind the desk, the papers so cover the desk that the fact that it is wooden is hidden. My experience of the desk includes shopping for it, moving it from house to house as my husband and I journeyed across the country, and spending many hours sitting at it to use the computer to write. Your experience of my desk would clearly be different.

Of course, nurses are seldom interested in describing experiences with such concrete items. What does interest us is the experience patients and nurses have of health, illness, and treatment. Sitting in a waiting room is very different for an anxious husband, for a woman waiting to be told the results of her breast biopsy, or for the nurse who enters the room many times each day of each week to invite patients to join her in the treatment rooms. Understanding patients' experiences may guide nurses to interact in ways that may differ from people who lack that understanding.

Phenomenological methodology, which seeks to understand another's experience, is ideally suited to the research of nursing care. Nurse theorists since Nightingale (1969) have discussed the need to understand patients' perceived needs in order to meet those needs effectively. The meanings that patients attribute to their experiences help create the needs they have and how these needs can best be met.

Because each patient is unique, individual patients must clarify what their perspectives and needs are. Only patients can reveal the meanings they create, and nurses cannot assume they understand patients' perspectives. Nurses can help only if they accurately understand patients' perspectives and their needs. Because action is based on meanings, common meanings between nurses and patients will provide the most effective base for helpful nurse-patient relationships. While practitioners need to understand the meanings that individual patients hold, understanding themes that go across patients (the outcome of phenomenological research) provides a useful guide to nurses as they seek to understand the individual's perspective. Understanding these common themes may be a useful beginning for assessment. In addition, knowing about common themes might make nurses more alert to issues that are alluded to by patients who may not be very clear or direct in their discussions.

Hermeneutic phenomenology is a research method based on phenomenological philosophy. The notion of hermeneutic phenomenology, first presented by Husserl and Dilthey, was changed significantly by Heidegger and Gadamer. Whereas Husserl and Dilthey were interested in learning about or understanding the structure of the *life-world* or lived experience, Heidegger expanded this definition of hermeneutics to include three different ideas. His first definition of hermeneutics is the process by which the "basic structures of Being . . . are made known." In the second definition, hermeneutics is the "working out of the conditions on which the possibility of any ontological investigation begins." Finally, Heidegger stated that hermeneutics is "an interpretation of Dasein's being" (Heidegger, 1962, pp. 37-38). As usual Heidegger is a little difficult to follow. *Dasein* is the German word for "being there." Heidegger used the term to refer to the human capacity to comprehend our own existence. Essentially what he is saying is that hermeneutics is: (a) the attempt to understand the phenomena of the world as they are presented to us (this is very close to the definition used by Husserl and Dilthey), (b) the attempt to understand how it is we go about understanding the world as it is presented to us, and (c) the attempt to understand being itself. That is, why is there something rather than nothing?

Gadamer (1989), in his analysis of Heidegger's work, made the argument that the second of these definitions is the appropriate concern of the human sciences. For him, hermeneutic phenomenology is research into how people go about understanding the world in which they live. His interest is not in the structure of phenomena but in how the phenomena are interpreted. Interpretation should then be the object of research (pp. 254-264).

What this means in practical terms is that the hermeneutic phenomenologist will study how people interpret their lives and make meaning of what they experience. Gadamer (1989) contended that hermeneutics is the study of *texts*. He used that term broadly to mean language. He included not only what people write down but also, more important, what they say and the symbolic activities in which they engage. He stated that to have a world is to have a language: "Our experience of the world is bound to language" (p. 448).

The other practical ramification of this definition of hermeneutic phenomenology is that the object of research is both language and the individual user of the language. Meaning takes place when a particular tradition—that is, the language of a group of people—is interpreted by a speaker. As Gadamer (1989) says, "It is literally more correct to say that language speaks us rather than we speak it" (p. 463). Thus the individual and the tradition must both be considered in hermeneutic phenomenology.

Hermeneutic phenomenological research bridges the traditional mind-body dichotomy that has long been debated by philosophers. Phenomenologists and existentialists argue that the mind and body (i.e., consciousness and physical existence) are not separate. The concept of intentionality expresses this unity by examining consciousness as "in the world" and always consciousness *of* something. Phenomenologists describe experience, where consciousness exists, rather than study emotions or thoughts in the abstract. For example, in our breast cancer study, this approach led us to ask women to describe what it was like for them to have breast cancer and experience its treatment rather than to ask them what they believe is important in health care in general. This philosophy has guided our investigation of the emotional needs of the physically ill with the aim of better understanding the impact of illness on people's lives and how nursing care can more effectively meet their needs.

HISTORICAL SKETCH

Although all research is based on a philosophy of science, or a worldview, this philosophy is not always articulated. Phenomenological philosophy is central to hermeneutic phenomenological research, and therefore, it is important to review both the philosophical assumptions of the approach and the phenomenological philosophy. Much has been written about philosophy of science; Suppe and Jacox (1985) provide a useful review of this topic and its relationship to nursing science. The semantic conception, worldview, or constructivist paradigm that is consistent with phenomenology includes a variety of assumptions that are important in hermeneutic phenomenological research. This includes the assumption that theory should be based on interpretations. Because interpretations are varied, there is no single reality. In addition, subjectivity is valued, context is important in explanations, biases need to be articulated, and ideas evolve and change over time.

Spiegelberg's (1984) book, *The Phenomenological Movement: A Historical Introduction,* is comprehensive and easy to read, and it presents important information about phenomenology. I shall provide a brief overview of the schools of philosophy and the schools of research that have developed from these schools of philosophy. I shall also discuss styles of conducting and presenting research within hermeneutic phenomenology, the approach we use.

Spiegelberg (1984) divided the phenomenological movement into three phases: the preparatory phase, the German phase, and the French phase. In an earlier article, I described these phases (Cohen, 1987). I will summarize them more briefly here. The *preparatory phase* involved two important people, Franz Brentano (1838-1917) and his student Carl Stumpf (1848-1936). Brentano's goal was to reform philosophy so that it could provide answers that organized religion could no longer supply. He also sought to make psychology truly scientific by basing it on descriptive psychology. Brentano's student, Stumpf, founded experimental phenomenology, which uses experimentation to discover the connections between the elements of what is being perceived. For example, he conducted experiments to study the psychological effects of sounds, including the influences of experiences (Stumpf, 1890/1912).

The next phase, the *German phase,* included both Edmund Husserl (1859-1938) and his student Martin Heidegger (1889-1976). Husserl is the central figure in the development of the phenomenological movement. It is referred to as a movement to note that the ideas involved in the philosophy have changed considerably—both across philosophers and within philosophers. This is also true of Husserl, whose ideas changed considerably over his career. Husserl's ideas included phenomenological reduction, also called *eidetic reduction* or *bracketing. Eidetic* is the adjective of *eidos,* Plato's alternative term for Idea (Form), which Husserl used to designate universal essences. It refers to a reduction from particular facts to general essences. Husserl used the mathematical metaphor of bracketing, meaning to bracket out one's prejudices and personal commitments, to understand meanings as they are for those describing the experiences. Other important concepts emerged in Husserl's work. These include the notion of *intersubjectivity,* which refers to a plurality of subjectivities who make up a community sharing a common world. *Life-world (Lebenswelt),* the world of lived experience, is another central concept found in Husserl's unpublished manuscripts.

The world of everyday experience is not immediately accessible to us in our "natural attitude." The natural is what is original and prior to critical or theoretical reflection. We take what is commonplace so much for granted that we often fail to notice it, and, therefore, phenomenological study is required.

Heidegger was Husserl's assistant for a time. He was primarily concerned with Being and with time (because Being is temporal). The two men seem to have lost contact later in Husserl's career, and much has been written about Heidegger's Nazi involvement and the fact that he did nothing to help Husserl (a Jew) during his retirement years. Phenomenology in Germany ended for all practical purposes with the Nazi years.

The third phase, the *French phase,* began when Husserl's papers were moved to Louvain shortly after his death. The key figures in this phase were Gabriel Marcel (1889-1973), Jean-Paul Sartre (1905-1980), and Maurice Merleau-Ponty (1908-1961). At the same time that phenomenological philosophies were developing, *Daseinanalyse,* or the existential-analytic movement, was developing among therapists.

These philosophical views of phenomenology were also used to develop research traditions in a number of disciplines, including nursing, which will be discussed later in this chapter. Hermeneutics or interpretive research has become a method used by a number of different disciplines, including sociologists such as Denzin, educators such as van Manen, and anthropologists such as Geertz. What sets hermeneutic phenomenology apart from these other hermeneutic approaches is the tradition of looking at a phenomenon, a single kind of human experience, rather than a social process or structure or a culture. Phenomenologists ask particular kinds of questions, such as our questions about dying and grief (Steeves), growing old (Kahn), and having cancer and its treatment (Cohen). We ask about how people interpret these experiences. Culture and social process may be parts of those experiences, but they are not the objects of interest, as they are in questions asked by sociologists and anthropologists. Phenomenology is different from grounded theory and ethnography. Whereas phenomenologists focus on questions of the meaning of experience, grounded theorists study social processes, and ethnographers are interested in understanding cultures and traditions.

Just as grounded theorists and ethnographers may be doing hermeneutic or interpretive research, a hermeneutic phenomenologist may borrow fieldwork techniques from both. For instance, in many places in the following chapters, techniques for participant observation, interviewing, and even sampling may sound like methods anthropologists might use in the field. But that does not mean we are describing ethnography. Our questions are not ethnographic questions, and our findings will not be ethnographic findings. But anthropologists have been conducting and writing about fieldwork for a long time, and there is no reason for us to ignore what they have learned about collecting data. What is important are philosophical matches or inconsistencies and doing rigorous research that will answer the questions that are important to nurses.

Current phenomenological research in nursing has been most influenced by Husserl, Heidegger, and the Dutch phenomenologists (Cohen & Omery, 1994). Husserl's eidetic or descriptive phenomenology has been influential because the Duquesne school of phenomenology is based on his philosophy. Giorgi, Colaizzi, Fischer, and van Kaam are the researchers from this school who are most often cited in nursing research. Heidegger's phenomenology has guided the school referred to as Heideggerian hermeneutics and interpretive phenomenology (Benner, 1984, 1994; Benner & Wrubel, 1989; Diekelmann, Allen, & Tanner, 1989). The Dutch phenomenology of the Utrecht School, including such scholars as Langeveld, Buitedijk, and Linschoten, has also been translated and applied to nursing research. Barritt, Beekman, Bleeker, and Mulderij (1983, 1984) and van Manen (1994) have written particularly clear and helpful texts describing Dutch phenomenology and its use in empirical research in education. This approach is also labeled hermeneutic phenomenology and is very similar to what we are presenting.

Differences exist among these traditions. The Duquesne researchers focus on eidetic description, those using Heideggerian hermeneutics focus on interpretation, and the hermeneutic phenomenological approach combines features of descriptive and interpretive phenomenology. Because individual researchers and schools of researchers have applied the philosophy and used variations in methods and forms of reporting, there is more variety in the use of these methods than this description might imply.

Phenomenologists and existentialists whose philosophies have guided our research include especially the Dutch phenomenology of the Utrecht School and also the work of Husserl, Sartre, Merleau-Ponty, and members of the existential-analytic movement of Daseinanalyse, including Binswanger, Ellenberger, and May.

LANGUAGE

Phenomenologists pay a good deal of attention to language. The meaning of words is important to think about because language is a primary way we express our meanings. Many words have taken on connotations that are not necessarily inherent in their meaning. Several key concepts have already been discussed in the context of the historical movement of phenomenological philosophy. The following is a list of additional words the definitions of which are important to hermeneutic phenomenological research, which is also referred to as the Utrecht School. These words are listed alphabetically after hermeneutic phenomenology.

Hermeneutic phenomenology is the label we use for our approach. The hermeneutic phenomenological method, or simply phenomenology, is also used interchangeably to avoid the lengthy label. The *hermeneutic* part of the label refers to the interpretation that accompanies description in our method. *The Oxford English Dictionary* (Brown, 1993) defines *hermeneutic* as "the branch of knowledge that deals with (theories of) interpretation, esp. of Scripture" (p. 1223). The word derives from the Greek verb meaning to interpret *(hermeneuo)*, which is derived from the name of the Greek god Hermes, who interpreted and conveyed messages from the gods to mortals (Mavromataki, 1997).

Literature on interpretation may have begun with the Rabbinic literature, which included various lists of hermeneutic principles (Hillel had 7 hermeneutic principles, Rabbi Yishmael had 13, and Rabbi Eliezer the son of Rabbi Yose HaGelili had 32). However, there have been many approaches used, and even the list of 613 principles compiled by Rabbi Meir Loeb ben Yehiel Michal was not an exhaustive list of all approaches found in Talmudic literature (Steinsaltz, 1989). Some of these Talmudic principles apply only to interpretation of the Bible, such as the principle of *superfluity* (p. 152), which is based on the assumption that every word of the Torah (the Written and Oral Law, including the Pentateuch) is precise and therefore significant. Although informants' words are important, there is no assumption in our research that every word is necessarily precise. However, other principles do apply to our research, such as "something learned from its context" (p. 151). Statements can be interpreted from the context in which they appear.

Empirical is defined in *The Oxford English Dictionary* (Brown, 1993) as "based on, guided by, or employing observation and experiment rather than theory and derived from or verifiable by experience" (p. 809). This is distinct from the philosophy of *empiricism*, which is defined as "the doctrine or theory that all knowledge is derived from sense-experience" (p. 809). Although the logical positivists and post-positivists often claim the word *empirical*, it actually applies as much to phenomenological research because phenomenologists study experience based on observation rather than theory.

Human science is a label that comes from the translation of the German word *geisteswissenschaften*, which refers to the social sciences and humanities as opposed to the natural sciences. Husserl is credited with being the first to search systematically for an adequate scientific foundation for geisteswissenschaften (Spiegelberg, 1984).

Intentionality means "directed toward something." Consciousness (awareness) is in the world and is always intentional; that is, it is always consciousness *of* something. Therefore, the study of experience reveals consciousness.

Phenomenological research was described earlier as the study of the meaning of experience. Research in which informants are asked to respond to a questionnaire and to write responses to some open-ended questions is qualitative but not phenomenological. In addition, other methods such as phenomenology, grounded theory, or ethnography are also qualitative. So although it is true that phenomenological research is qualitative, the word *qualitative* is general, with a wider meaning. An additional label to describe hermeneutic phenomenological research is *naturalistic*. Because the term *qualitative* includes more research methods than does the term *naturalistic*, the former has the disadvantage of being less specific. There are both similarities and differences among naturalistic and qualitative methods, and perhaps making distinctions among these methods by using their precise labels is most useful. Another useful distinction is that *naturalistic* refers to the way data are collected, *ethnographic* refers to the way data will be used, which is to describe cultures, and, finally, *phenomenological* refers to the way data are analyzed and to the philosophical underpinnings of the approach.

Reliability and *validity* are words that carry with them ideas from the logical positivists, which is the primary reason many phenomenologists object to them. They argue for use of words such as *trustworthiness* and *accuracy* to convey these ideas. However, others argue that the concepts behind these words apply equally well to the standards of quality important to all research and that they can be redefined or translated to fit phenomenological research.

Saturation is an example of language developed by those who used grounded theory methodology. The word refers to the idea that researchers have obtained enough data to have a complete description of the experience being studied. It is a useful concept, although the most orthodox researchers may criticize borrowing the language of another research tradition. We are not arguing against borrowing language when it is appropriate, and this concept is appropriate to hermeneutic phenomenological research, but we do caution that the connotations that come with the language should be considered.

Science is a word derived from the Latin *scientia,* meaning "knowledge," and it is defined as "knowledge acquired by study" (Brown, 1993, p. 2717). It is often used to mean the study of the physical universe. However, as with the word empirical, this narrowing of the definition seems unjustified.

Subjects is a word seldom used by phenomenologists. It conjures up the notion of subjects and objects and also does not give the connotation of partnership that is important to phenomenological research. Those who participate in phenomenological research are perhaps more appropriately called informants, because they inform us about their experience.

This research methodology involves in-depth interviews, analysis of these interviews, and descriptions of the key elements of experience. Phenomenological research is gaining recognition but is still relatively new to nurse researchers.

This chapter has described the historically important philosophical bases for the hermeneutic phenomenological approach and some of the key concepts in the method. The next chapter will provide an overview of writing the research proposal. Although it is not the first step in beginning a project, the process of writing a proposal provides an overview of the entire research process.

2

WRITING THE PROPOSAL

MARLENE Z. COHEN

The proposal writing process is presented in this chapter because understanding the process provides an overview of what is involved in a phenomenological research project. See Chapter 3 for a discussion on getting started, because writing a proposal is not the first step in any research process.

Hermeneutic phenomenological research has the advantage of being less dependent on expensive technology than other methods. The researcher does, however, need time. Some of the time-consuming tasks (such as transcription of audiotape-recorded interviews) can be done by others if funding is available. Much of the work—for example, the analysis—is time-consuming and cannot be delegated to others. Obtaining funding for salary (i.e., time) is also very helpful.

Funding can be obtained from a variety of sources depending on the expertise of the researcher and the amount of money sought. This chapter will discuss the continuum of funding sources, from small local funds to large federal and other grants. Knowing the audience, that is, who the reviewers are, is a crucial first step. These same points apply to proposals written for purposes other than obtaining money, such as theses, dissertations, or institutional review board proposals.

Issues likely to arise in constructing a proposal will be discussed, such as the need for pilot data for larger (such as National Institutes of Health, or NIH) proposals. Differences between the hermeneutic phenomenological approach and other research methods and how these can be reframed for the reviewers will also be discussed. For example, the importance of including a detailed method section for proposals that are requesting large amounts of money and ways to illustrate the approach to data analysis will be discussed.

WRITING EFFECTIVE PROPOSALS

Writing an effective proposal is very much like gaining entry for research, a task with which phenomenologists are very familiar. It is important to understand the purpose of the proposal and to know what the reviewer will be looking for. A basic need is to answer the questions in the reviewer's mind, and these questions vary somewhat depending on the type of proposal.

Proposals can be thought of as falling along a continuum. The first type of proposal likely to be written is the proposal students need to write for a class project, a thesis, or dissertation research. Early postgraduate work may involve applying for internal funding from employers. External funding is most often sought at the other end of this continuum, although mechanisms for external funding for students and those early in their careers also exist (Tripp-Reimer & Cohen, 1991). Proposals for external funding could be either for small grants or for larger grants.

Although a complete proposal for a larger grant cannot be written until one conducts a small pilot study, it is useful to begin with an understanding of the sections of a proposal and the gestalt sought. The format or a proposal depends on its purpose, who will be reading it, and the guidelines that the agency has developed; however, six sections are most commonly required. The labels for the headings may well vary, but the content will be similar.

1. *Abstract:* The abstract is an overview used to orient the reviewer to the project. Although it is placed at the beginning of the proposal, it is usually the last section to be written. The abstract should include a brief but complete summary of what is in the proposal. Be sure to include the *significance* of the research, discussing why it is important to do this study. How does the literature show this is an important problem? Discuss the *purpose* of the study, the *methods,* the *sample,* and the *outcome* of the research. Aim for one or two sentences about each of these five topics, depending on the length allowed for the abstract.

2. *Specific aims:* This is the heart and essence of the proposal, and although it comes first in many proposals, this section most often must be revised after the literature has been examined and the methods have been described in more detail. The specific aims are focused, well defined, and explicit. They let the reviewer know what will be accomplished in terms of the objectives of the project, not the procedures. This should be a brief section, written in simple sentences that describe what will be done, to whom, why, and where. If there are a series of objectives, arrange them logically in order of importance or in the sequence in which they will be accomplished.

An example of specific aims was published in Tripp-Reimer and Cohen (1991, p. 248). This phenomenological research proposal included six specific aims:

1. Obtain descriptions of patients' experiences of their hospitalization for surgery and the nursing care they received.

2. Obtain descriptions of nurses' perceptions of these same patients' experiences of their hospitalization for surgery and the nursing care they received.

3. Analyze and present these descriptions using phenomenological methods (Barritt et al., 1983).

4. Identify patients' perceived priority needs and concerns after surgery and how nurses were helpful or not helpful to them.

5. Identify nurses' priority concerns for these postoperative patients.

6. Compare patients' and nurses' priorities.

3. Significance: This section in an NIH proposal is the literature review. A misconception about phenomenological research is that the researcher begins the project with no review of the literature. Although the researcher ought not to suggest ideas to informants in the interviews, the reality is that no one will allow research to be conducted today without a proposal. This section builds a case for why the study is needed. This is done by reviewing and critiquing classic and current literature on the topic and closely related topics. This section would also include any prior research the applicant has conducted that shows why this study is needed and how it fits with what is known and unknown about this topic. This section should lead the reader to understand that the proposed research will fill an important gap in our knowledge.

4. Methods: The methods sections need to be written in as much detail as possible to convince reviewers that the project is feasible and that the researcher knows what needs to be done. The length of this section of the proposal depends on prior research (a small pilot study). There are four major sections:

   A. *Design:* Briefly describe the design of the study (in our case it will be the hermeneutic phenomenological approach). In smaller proposals (which are likely to be shorter and have budgets requesting less money), labeling the design and very briefly describing it will be enough detail. Larger (such as NIH) proposals will require more detail.

   B. *Sample:* Tell as much as you know about the informants at this point, and what characteristics they need to have to be included. For example, in our breast cancer study, women who had had mastectomies were included, and women who did not speak English were excluded. Proposals for larger grants require letters of support from people who will help you find your informants and perhaps information about the agencies from which informants will be obtained. This is to ensure the reviewers that there will be enough people who fit your criteria for you to complete your project in the time you have allotted.

   C. *Procedures:* Explain exactly how, when, where, and with whom you will collect your data and what form the data will take: verbatim transcriptions of audiotape-recorded interviews, fieldnotes, and/or existing documents.

   D. *Data analysis:* Describe how you will manage, sort, categorize, and reduce your data (see Chapter 7). Providing an example from your pilot study or prior research is often helpful.

5. Consent form: The format for consent forms varies with each institutional review board (IRB). (Chapter 4 provides more detail about IRBs.)

Many institutions have developed standards or guidelines for consent forms to be used for research in that setting. It is very important to learn about what is used in the setting from which you will seek informants. Different consent forms may well be needed for a study that involves obtaining informants from more than one institution.

The consent form is usually part of a research proposal. There is a core of standard information, including a clear statement that what is proposed is research; the purpose of the research; how people are selected for inclusion; an explanation of all procedures, risks, and benefits; alternatives to participating; assurance of anonymity and confidentiality; the offer to answer questions; and the option to withdraw. A slightly edited example from our breast cancer study (Cohen et al., 1998) is found in Figure 2.1.

6. *References:* There are usually page limitations for the research proposal. The list of references is not usually included in these designated limitations. The references need to be both current and comprehensive to show you have a grasp of the current and classic literature on the topic.

ISSUES TO CONSIDER IN PROPOSAL WRITING

In determining how to write the proposal, one question is how likely the reviewers are to be familiar with phenomenological research. Wise students construct their thesis or dissertation committee (those who will be reviewing their proposal) with members who know this method or at least are open to the approach. Having a methodological expert on the committee will be extremely useful. In any case, the project, thesis, or dissertation proposal needs to convince the faculty members that the student knows enough about the topic and method to be able to conduct the research. When proposals are written to obtain funding, reviewers must be convinced both that the proposal writer knows enough about the topic and method to be able to conduct the research and that the research results will be worth the investment of their money. Internal funders are likely to consider the initial funding as an investment in developing the researcher's career. External agencies are more likely to be concerned with the substantive contribution the research will make to the topic or area being studied.

TITLE:	The experience of breast cancer: Nursing implications
DEPARTMENT:	Nursing
PRINCIPAL INVESTIGATOR:	Marlene Zichi Cohen, RN, PhD
24 HOUR PHONE: (EMERGENCY)	

PURPOSE: You have been asked to participate in this study because you have been recently diagnosed with breast cancer. The purpose of this research is to describe and compare the experiences of women with breast cancer in order to develop better ways for nurses to help them.

PROCEDURE: In an interview with a nurse you will be asked some general background information and then will be asked general questions about what it is like for you to have breast cancer. The interview, which will last approximately one hour, will be tape-recorded, transcribed word for word, and analyzed for common content. No information that identifies you will be included on the written copy of your interview. Your name and the names of others you mention will be replaced by a code. We may contact you to verify our analysis and will provide you with a copy of our results at the end of the study if you would like them.

RISKS: You may experience some inconvenience due to the time involved in being interviewed. You may feel uncomfortable discussing this sensitive topic. Your participation will not impact your medical treatment.

BENEFITS: Possible benefits for you include the value of reflecting on your experiences. You will have the opportunity to discuss this topic with an interested nurse. You may also experience some satisfaction from participating in this study that may help determine the most useful way for nurses to provide care to meet breast cancer patients' needs.

ALTERNATIVES: The alternative to participating in this research is not to be interviewed. You are free to withhold any information you prefer not to discuss and can refuse to answer any questions we ask. You can participate in the first interview and refuse to talk at later times.

FIGURE 2.1. Patients' Informed Consent Form

CONFIDENTIALITY: Your medical records will not be looked at for this study. The confidentiality of your interview will be maintained by the investigators and the Research Committee (IRB). Tapes will be stored until the end of the study and then erased. In the unlikely event that you discuss harming yourself or others, we will maintain confidentiality only to the extent allowable by law.

OFFER TO ANSWER QUESTIONS: This research will not affect your treatment in any way. Any questions or concerns which you may have about this research study may be reported to Marlene Z. Cohen, RN, PhD,[followed by office address and telephone number] or the Institutional Review Board (Research Committee) [followed by office address and telephone number]

COERCION AND WITHDRAWAL STATEMENT: Your decision whether or not to participate will not interfere with your future care at this institution. If you decide to participate, you are free to withdraw your consent and to discontinue participation at any time.

PHYSICAL INJURY STATEMENT: In the highly unlikely event that you require medical treatment as a result of physical injury arising from your participation in this study, the financial responsibility for such will be yours.

FINANCIAL RESPONSIBILITY STATEMENT: There is no cost to you from participating in this research.

NEW INFORMATION: Any new information that is developed during the course of research which may relate to your willingness to continue or discontinue participation in this study will be provided to you.

AGREEMENT: Your signature indicates that you have decided to participate having read the information provided above.

_____

Signature of Participant

_____

Signature of Witness

_____

Date

Good writing standards should be applied to proposal writing. Proposals need to be written in the future tense, because they are describing work that *will be* conducted. Using the language of the funder is important and demonstrates the importance of knowing the audience. It is wise to write the proposal using as much of the reviewer's language as possible.

If the language the funder or agency requires does not quite fit the hermeneutic phenomenological method, it may be useful to give an explanation. For example, I submitted a protocol to the IRB of the comprehensive cancer center where the patients I would be interviewing had their bone marrow transplantation. Because this IRB most often reviewed proposals for clinical trials of drugs, the format it used included topics that did not apply to phenomenological research. These items included, for example, "drug information and staging criteria." Because the reviewers of these protocols look for this information in each protocol, I included these headings and wrote under them "not applicable." Similarly, for other items, the commonly used headings were included with an explanation. For the section "Statistical Considerations," I wrote, "Qualitative analysis of data will be employed," and a detailed discussion of analysis was included in another section of the proposal.

Write proposals in a positive way. That is, it is more useful to talk about what you will be doing instead of what you will not be doing. For example, you would talk about obtaining a description, rather than say you will not be testing hypotheses, unless you are "reframing" for an audience who may not understand phenomenological methods.

Formatting for easy reading is also helpful. Subheadings may help to draw the reviewer to the different sections. A good impression is not made if a proposal contains spelling or other errors. Correct citations and consistent format for references are also important. The purpose of the reference list is to allow reviewers to know and find the sources to which you refer. That means unpublished sources are not very useful and ought to be avoided. Secondary references should also be avoided if at all possible, because the secondary author may well have incorrectly interpreted the original author's work.

When justifying why something will or will not be done, it is most useful to provide scientific reasons. No project is perfect, and no researcher ever has all the time and money to do everything that might be desired.

For example, it is better to write about why what you are doing will attain your goals rather than to write that the number of informants is determined by time or funding constraints.

Proposals need to contain enough detail to show that both the topic and approach have been well thought out. Methods should be described in detail. For student and small proposals, reading the literature may provide sufficient detail. Large proposals will more likely require conducting a pilot study. The reality for all research is that initial plans seldom, if ever, can be implemented without alteration. In addition, aspects of research that are less familiar to reviewers may need to be illustrated with a concrete example from a pilot study. For instance, in our research proposals, we have included examples of data analysis as well as examples of how we communicated as a team working at different sites.

The interview guide is an important detail to include in the proposal. IRBs, other reviewers, and sometimes informants want to know exactly what you will ask the informants in the interviews. It is not enough to say simply "unstructured interviews will be conducted." Interviewers will focus informants on the topic being studied in some way, and a brief interview guide helps to show how that will be done. For example, when studying the experience of critical care hospitalization, we asked, "What was it like for you to be in the intensive care unit?" We did not simply turn on the tape recorder and record whatever the patient wanted to talk about (Cohen, Craft, & Titler, 1988). Another example comes from the study of the experience of having surgery. One informant talked at some length about playing golf. I let this continue because I expected him to make a connection with his surgery. When he did not link the golf to his surgery, I asked him how golf was connected to his surgery. He told me it was not related, he just liked to talk about golf. Returning informants to the interview topic is sometimes needed.

BUDGET PROJECTIONS

Budget is an important aspect to consider when writing a proposal. Reviewers will want to see a realistic budget. Therefore, drastic over- or underestimations of projected costs may only impress on the reviewer that the proposal writer does not have a good understanding of what is involved in the proposed research project.

Salary is, of course, a major expense and is likely to be included in larger proposals. Phenomenological research is time-consuming. Regardless of whether or not an investigator's salary is funded, it may also be useful to seek funding for graduate student research assistants (RAs). These RAs can assist with the time-consuming aspects of the research and obtain valuable learning from their involvement.

There are a variety of aspects of the research that can be delegated to RAs. In hermeneutic phenomenological research, RAs can transcribe tape-recorded interviews. If a transcriptionist has been hired, RAs can verify the accuracy of the transcripts. They can also assist with doing literature searches and copying articles. With proper preparation and supervision, RAs can conduct interviews. They can also assist with various aspects of data management, including matching fieldnotes with interviews and keeping copies of documents available. And finally, they can assist with manuscript preparation and should be coauthors if their contributions are sufficient to justify authorship.

It is, of course, important to remember that the research assistantship is a learning experience. Some thought should be given to the level of the RA's expertise, the value of the tasks in learning how to conduct good research, and the need for supervision. Gift, Creasia, and Parker (1991) provided a comprehensive overview of the effective use of RAs.

Transcription is an important, tedious task. When seeking a transcriptionist, it may be useful to pay a bit more for someone with transciption skills and experience. In any case, when estimating the cost of a transcriptionist, keep in mind that verbatim transcription requires 3 to 4 hours of typing per hour of tape.

Although not much equipment is needed for phenomenological research, some things are needed, and these will be described in the next chapter. These items can be included in the budget depending on the amount of money available from the funding agency. Investing in a tape recorder with a good microphone and good quality recording tapes is a worthwhile expense. The quality of recording greatly influences the time needed for and the quality of transcription. You will also need batteries so remember to budget for them. Investing in a transcription machine with a foot pedal will be useful for both initial transcription and for reviewing the transcripts to ensure the accuracy of the transcription.

FUNDING FOR PHENOMENOLOGICAL RESEARCH

Many fine books and articles have been written about writing grants and proposals, and these may be useful to review. There is a common belief that grant reviewers will not fund a project that is completely phenomenological (or completely qualitative or naturalistic, for that matter). Cohen, Knafl, and Dzurec (1993) found this was not true when they asked qualitative researchers to send them pink sheets from qualitative research proposals. (Pink sheets is the label given to grant reviewers' critiques. These critiques were originally sent on pink paper. Although the paper is no longer this color, the label has remained.) A content analysis of these pink sheets revealed that good proposals are indeed funded, and several areas were important to the reviewers of these grants. These areas included a well-written qualitative grant proposal was one with a thoroughly developed statement of a significant, relevant problem for nursing. It addressed that problem using appropriate methods or combinations of methods that were described clearly, succinctly, and thoroughly with appropriate rationale. Reviewers said the problems presented should be based on an appropriate literature review, and it was useful to have the writer of the proposal describe how the study can be interpreted as valid and reliable (Cohen et al., 1993).

This chapter has reviewed writing grant proposals, including

- types of proposals
- the six most commonly required sections of grant proposals
- issues in proposal writing such as the reviewers' familiarity with the hermeneutic phenomenological approach, writing clearly and in a positive manner about what will be accomplished, and budgetary considerations

3

HOW TO START FIELDWORK

RICHARD H. STEEVES

The steps in carrying out any research project are not at all orderly. The chapter on proposal writing precedes this chapter on starting fieldwork because most beginning researchers believe it happens that way. One writes a proposal, then carries out that proposal as closely to the written word as possible. But the truth is that a researcher cannot write a full proposal without first spending at least a little time in the field to understand various aspects of experience. Sometimes, entry to the field is made not as a researcher but as a volunteer or in some other capacity, and, sometimes, entry into the field starts long before a research question is even imagined. For instance, I worked taking calls for hospices for several years before I began to collect data for my research with hospice patients. Researchers cannot anticipate the problems that may occur and, more important, cannot convince a funding agency that they will be able to accrue informants unless they already have access to the field site. In this chapter, I shall discuss choosing a field site, gaining access, maintaining access, and choosing what to take into the field.

Nurses conduct research in a variety of venues, but the two most common places and, arguably, the two most useful places are clinical settings and informants' homes. We are most interested in individuals who are or might become sick and need health care. Sometimes, the health care is only a potentiality, as in my study of elderly African Americans and Appalachians bereaved at the loss of a spouse; most of the informants did not seek or need health care. Sometimes, the clinic and the clinical workers are of prime interest, and the individual patients assume the position of being a potentiality. That is, one could be interested in how decisions are made and conflicts are resolved in a busy emergency department. The informants would all be workers in the emergency department. The long-range goal, however, would be to determine how the atmosphere in which care is delivered is created. Nurse researchers certainly could be interested in the interactions within and between professional groups. Our education and socialization usually does not allow our interest to rest there long.

CHOOSING A FIELD SITE

Most researchers, even first-time student researchers, are quite capable of choosing a field setting without much guidance. Researchers go to places and talk to people who have experiences that the researchers decide are of scientific interest. That is exactly as it should be. Each new generation of researchers defines what is appropriate for study. Handed-down orthodoxies are deadly for good science.

A myth that must be dispelled is that researchers are somehow advantaged by going to places about which they are completely ignorant. Even if researchers were capable of identifying such a place, why would they be the least interested in going there? Certainly, there is an appeal to exploring the unknown, but astronauts did not travel to the moon without learning all that could be known without being there. Ignorance has never helped a field researcher or scientist of any kind. This is not to say, however, that nurse researchers working in a setting where they have been or are presently clinicians is an advantage. Maintaining a separation of roles (the same people should generally not be both patients and informants for a nurse/researcher) presents some difficult problems. Unless nurses have complete control in selecting patients from a setting for whom they will provide care (a rare circumstance), the chance that an informant will be assigned to them as a patient is always present.

ACCESS TO CLINICAL SETTINGS

Understanding the structure of power and authority in a clinical setting is essential to successful fieldwork in that setting. The power structure can be simple and straightforward, as in a small clinic or office owned and operated by a single provider; or it can be Byzantine as in a large teaching hospital. Either way, it is necessary to understand as much as possible who makes which decisions. Sometimes, this may not be easy, given that it is convenient and useful for some managers to obfuscate the source of authority and thereby the culpability for certain kinds of decisions.

In a research project with bone marrow transplant patients (Steeves, 1992a) I completed some years ago, I was interested in following informants through their hospital stay. I talked with the nursing administration and the floor nurses on all three shifts. I explained my study to the medical division chair. A meeting was arranged with the chief resident and the remainder of the house staff. I thought I had access from the clinical staff and could begin to recruit patients. But I had forgotten the medical director of the outpatient clinic. Even though the patients were not seen by the outpatient staff once they were in the hospital, they were seen by this staff before admission and after discharge. The director of the outpatient clinic found out about my study, and the study was halted until I could verify the scientific merit of the study for him.

In my study of hospice caregivers of people with cancer, I learned the importance of some of the least powerful people, or at least those with less formal power than many others in the system. I had the permission and the cooperation of the formal leaders of the hospice, the director of nursing, the executive director, and the field nurses, but the people who were actually available by telephone on a daily basis were the clerks. These two women actually had a broad picture of the operations of the agency and kept track of all the admissions and discharges. To recruit informants, I needed to know about the admissions.

The clerks had little incentive to help me. Paying attention to each admission to determine if the caregiver met the criteria for my study was extra work, and they had little to gain by doing it. With professional staff, I could draw on the notion of the value of research for the profession. The responsibility of the clerks, however, was to ensure the smooth day-to-day operations of the agency. They had every reason to wish I would just go away and not bother them or the functioning of the agency. Yet it was these clerks who could most reliably locate the informants.

So I learned to spend time with the clerks. Not long periods of time—I would have been considered more of a nuisance that way—but a little time on frequent occasions. I made small talk and sometimes brought doughnuts for the break room (a research expense that cannot be charged to a grant). I needed them to like me, or at least not be able to ignore me altogether or actively dislike me. I was hoping they would connect my face with the request to scan all new admissions for certain characteristics.

Employees want their bosses to like them; bosses want their employees to be happy; students want their teachers to notice them in a favorable way. The business of the world runs on this Lacanian notion of our ability to behold our humanity in the gaze of another. Most of the time, an informal and unspoken but felt commitment is what allows the work of the world to be accomplished.

Sometimes, access to informants is more costly than small talk and doughnuts. In my study of bone marrow transplant patients (Steeves, 1992a), I wanted to do more than talk with the patients; I was interested in studying the unit as well. In this unit, each patient was admitted under one of several research protocols. In a great many, perhaps most health care delivery systems, patients are "owned" by somebody. Usually, the owner is an attending physician. A researcher cannot approach a patient, cannot even learn salient details about a patient, without the permission of the attending physician. From the physician's point of view, this makes sense. The patient is where he or she is (in the hospital or clinic, etc.) because of a relationship with a physician. This relationship carries with it a reasonable expectation of privacy; patients would expect physicians not to give their names or details about them to anyone else. Thus, a researcher needs to approach most potential informants in health care settings through the attending physician.

But in the case of the bone marrow transplant inpatient unit where I sought informants, the patients were admitted to a research protocol, not to a particular attending physician. The attending physician began to follow the patient after the patient was admitted to a particular protocol. Therefore, obtaining access to a patient meant approaching the Principal Investigator (PI) for the research protocol under which the patient was to be admitted.

I met with the PI for a protocol that would give me access to patients and the unit, explained my study, and was eventually given permission to start my study. During the meeting with the PI, I learned a great deal about the unit and why it was run the way it was run. The PI was concerned that I should understand how very sick the patients were at times and how difficult talking with them would be during parts of their treatment. She offered me a chance to be on the unit and see and talk to the patients before I began my study formally. I could be a data collector for her study protocol.

The intent of the PI was certainly not to make me pay with free labor for the privilege of having access to patients. This was not a quid pro quo arrangement. But she understood that I did not want to be an outsider on the unit and with the staff. Also, she wanted to ensure that I would not be so inexperienced that I would be a possible source of harm (in terms of spreading infection and psychological trauma). So she set me to work. I worked part-time for several months before I began to collect data on my own study. The lesson I learned from these experiences was that I must learn as much as I possibly can about the social world in which I am to collect data, by any means that are presented to me.

VISITING PEOPLE IN THEIR HOMES

In most people's lives, there is no social category for researcher. That is, generally, people know how to behave with and toward others in their environment based on what category that other falls into. The variety of people who visit homes is rather limited: relatives, friends, neighbors, salespeople, meter readers, and repair people. Usually our choices are straightforward. Friends who come for dinner are not treated the same as the plumber. Occasionally, there is awkwardness when a friend is hired to repair the plumbing, but generally the categories are easy to maintain and are helpful in navigating social situations.

Most people, however, do not have researchers visit their homes. When researchers do arrive, therefore, no social rules governing behavior of researchers or informants exist. In the bereavement study, I visited informants as a hospice volunteer. This did not work well. Hospice volunteers generally visit the house of a dying person for a set period of time to accomplish a task that is agreed on in advance. Volunteers sit with dying people or read to them so the primary caregiver can rest or run errands. Volunteers drive family members who cannot drive themselves; they cut firewood or mow the lawn. I could have done all these things as a researcher acting as a volunteer, and in many cases I did. But this work interfered with the work I needed to do as a researcher. Participant observation could sometimes be accomplished as a volunteer, but the interviews and my attendance at churches and parties did not fit with the social role of a volunteer. Thus, rarely was I a hospice volunteer in my mind and, I would imagine, in the minds of my informants. I did not primarily visit to help out. I wanted to talk, or rather I wanted to listen as they talked. Also, it should be made clear that misrepresentation of oneself is never acceptable. Gaining access to a social situation as a volunteer or in any other social role, then using that access to collect data as a participant observer, is ethically wrong when informants have not been completely informed about (and consented to) the researcher's purpose for being there.

On occasion, I was treated more as a meter reader than anything else. One woman, who owned and operated a large cattle farm, tolerated me because she had agreed to participate in the study. But she expected me to come, ask my questions as efficiently as possible, and leave. Because I really did not have a set of questions but was interested in her experiences, this was not a good situation for me. In her opinion, I was a man who worked for the hospice and should just do my job and get on with it.

Most of the time, I was closer to the social category appropriate for a neighbor than to anything else. I was not a friend. I was not someone who was invited to dinner with my family or to a movie or to come over and watch a ball game. On the few occasions when I was invited to such friendly events, I politely declined. I was someone who dropped by on an afternoon for a talk; I could be counted on to show up for the important events, such as funerals, weddings, and anniversaries. Most important, I was a listener and not a gossip. Informants could expect my opinions on the weather and the national news but not on a mutual acquaintance or another neighbor. I tried to be a good neighbor.

Being a good neighbor requires some learning in each neighborhood. Some examples might be illustrative. Mildred, an informant in the bereavement study, let me know early in my visits what was expected of me. I was to bring food, usually fruit. She was in her 80s, lived in a few rooms of the cluttered, unpainted, clapboard house she and her husband had built themselves, and subsisted on her share of her dead husband's minimum Social Security. She could not see well enough to drive, so her daughter hid the keys to her truck. Mildred knew where the keys were but had acquiesced to the fact that she could not drive while refusing to admit it to her family.

Because she could not drive to the grocery store and would not have much money to spend if she could, she did not have perishables in her house. I was expected to bring bananas, or oranges, or occasionally a pineapple. Naturally, she did not ask me outright to bring her fruit. She merely mentioned that a neighbor sometimes brought her fruit and how much she appreciated it.

As payback, Mildred cooked for me. At first, I thought this was a terrible idea. I did not want to share the small sustenance she had for herself. But I discovered this was an occasion for Mildred to eat. That is, she was not hungry often and was beginning to think it was too much of a bother to cook. I was afraid she would begin to lose weight and strength. When I came to lunch, she would cook and eat with me. It became clear that on many occasions, this was her only meal of the day. I could hardly refuse, even though, despite my southern upbringing, I have never cared for greens cooked with a ham hock.

Bob Morris had a different set of expectations. His wife was dying with multiple myeloma, or that is what her doctor and the hospice believed. Bob did not believe it, and 2½ years later, he seemed to be right. But Bob had hospice care for his wife and signed up for my study. When I was visiting, Bob spent almost no time in the house. He was a farmer and had over 120 head of cattle, so he always had outside work to do. His youngest daughter had moved back home and was taking care of her mother. Bob could have hired a farmhand or sold off the cattle, but he did not want to be in the house tending to his sick wife.

As far as Bob was concerned, neighbors did not come to sit and talk. They talked, but they talked out in the barn or in the shed or during the drive to a distant pasture. Neighbors did not show up with a tape recorder and certainly would not expect him to stop work to have his conversation recorded. We welded braces on a trailer for his cows; we repaired fences and put new brake shoes on his tractor. All the time, I tried to remember what he was telling me so I could write it down later. This is not to say that there was not a considerable amount of time leaning against a fence post, sitting on a tractor tire, or riding in the pickup truck just talking. But the talking needed to be in the context of work for Bob to be comfortable with it.

Sometimes, it was difficult to understand how a neighbor should act. Jessie was a fellow in his late 60s caring for his wife, who was dying of breast cancer. Jessie's family had lived in the Blue Ridge Mountains for two centuries, and I was just beginning to learn how neighbors should behave in his culture.

On a Saturday afternoon, Jessie invited me to an anniversary party for friends, family, church people, and neighbors. I bought a small anniversary gift the day before and wrapped it in silver paper. I drove out a little early to the house wearing a tie but no jacket. It was summer, and very few people wear jackets in my part of the world on a summer afternoon. I was not sure about the tie, so I sat in the car and waited to see a few others go into the house. No one was wearing a tie, so I took mine off and left it in the car.

But when I entered with my gift in hand, I realized I had made a mistake. There was no table piled with gifts, and no one made an effort to take my gift or show me where to put it. I was the only one who had brought a gift. I was greeted warmly and politely anyway and shown into the dining room where there was a "money tree." This was a new experience for me. Nailed to a stand pointing up like a Christmas tree was a branch from a hardwood tree without its leaves. In the place where the leaves would be was money, $10 or $20 bills, sometimes just a dollar, clipped on with a clothespin. I left my present beside the tree, but I also clipped a $5 bill (all I had) to a branch and made a mental note about how good neighbors behave in Jessie's neighborhood.

Generally speaking, learning how to talk and act like a good neighbor, including how to give and work and eat, is the key to collecting data in informants' homes.

THE BAG: TAKING EQUIPMENT TO THE FIELD

Some qualitative researchers eschew technology (Lincoln & Guba, 1985) and prefer not to tape-record interviews. The argument is that the tape recorder is intrusive enough to change the quality of the data. The counterargument is that after the first few minutes, informants seem to ignore the tape recorder all together. But it is difficult to deny the effect of taping. Although it is true that informants ignore the little machine after a few minutes, the rules and atmosphere for the interview have been established by that time. When one is conducting hermeneutic phenomenological research, however, the atmosphere and rules for the interview established by the presence of a tape recorder are not necessarily unhelpful and may indeed be necessary to the process. As pointed out earlier, the hermeneutic phenomenological researcher is gathering stories, and it is acknowledged that these stories are artifacts, a kind of fiction, created for the telling. The presence of a tape recorder may help to establish that the informant is creating something of importance to the researcher. But, of course, this is guesswork; it is difficult to tell what an informant thinks about a tape recorder without asking, and asking such a question might cause the kind of reflexivity that inhibits discourse of any kind. In the end, it seems most useful to tape-record interviews and have a somewhat accurate representation of the data for analysis. Also tape-recording an interview means that the researcher does not have to take extensive notes and therefore may be more involved in the discourse.

The following discussion may seem obvious to some but may offer some protection from unnecessary hassles for the beginning fieldworker. The following are lessons learned from frustration and error because no one told me how to pack for the field.

A camera bag, although a little expensive, works well for packing the equipment necessary for fieldwork. A backpack, nylon briefcase, or conference bag works almost as well but often does not have the padding and the numerous little pouches a camera bag has. Of course, camera bags are prime targets if you will be someplace where you might be robbed. The camera bag should contain the following:

1. Tape recorder

2. Microphones

3. Tapes

4. Batteries

5. Towel

6. Hardbacked notebook

7. Colored pens

The tape recorder itself need not be terribly expensive. Perhaps the cheapest one available would not be a good investment, but the tape recorders designed for recording music are not necessary. The nuances of sound are not usually important in recording interviews, but noise and static can reduce the reliability of the transcripts and thus the quality of the study. Therefore, a good tape recorder is worth some investment. Soon the technology will be available to digitalize voice recording directly, and tapes will be played directly into computer programs. When that becomes the case, it will be important to ensure that the two technologies are compatible. If you will be transcribing the tapes yourself or if you hire a transcriptionist, make sure the transcription machine you have available and the tape recorder you use play the same size tape. Most tape recorders have a voice-activated system. That is, they begin to record only when a sound is sensed. This system does not work well for research interviews. Sometimes, the size of a pause in conversation will be important, and those data will be missing. But more important, the first syllable of a word after a pause will be missing. This is very frustrating for a transcriptionist, who is probably working by the hour and may be one of the most costly parts of the project. Turn off the voice-activated system.

Most tape recorders have a built-in microphone and a jack for plugging in an auxiliary microphone. For recording fieldnotes, when the tape recorder can be held up close to your mouth, the built-in microphone works well. In an informant's home, a directional microphone (fairly inexpensive) improves the quality of the sound considerably. Lapel microphones are also cheap and may be worth packing in your bag. Occasionally, an informant will have a very soft voice or a physiological problem with speech, and the lapel microphone is worth the intrusion it creates. The lapel microphone should be saved for special circumstances because the wire is usually short (longer ones are available at some stores) and the informant will have to either have the tape recorder in his/her lap as well as the microphone or be connected to a tape recorder placed on a nearby table. This creates the unavoidable and unpleasant feeling of being wired up.

Naturally, it is important to carry spare tapes. One cannot be sure how long an interview will last, and stopping a good interview because one is out of tape is very frustrating. Tapes and the small plastic cases they come in can become separated. It is important, therefore, to write all the pertinent information about the interview on the tape itself, as well as on the card that shows through the plastic case. Always choose to have more information on the tape rather than less. Double-checking records of data is so much easier when information is redundant in numerous places. Sixty-minute tapes are the upper limit on the reliability of batteries. A partially drained battery will pull a 90-minute tape at a rate that distorts the sound.

The tape recorder, the directional microphone, and the lapel microphone all require batteries. The bag should contain more than one spare of each size. Having a drained battery in the field is a real nuisance; therefore, a good policy is to change all the batteries on a regular schedule, once every 2 weeks, perhaps, if the interviews are long or the interview schedule is busy.

Carrying a towel in the camera case can be helpful. Only when you begin to tape conversations do you realize how selective the human ear is. We not only hear, but we listen and selectively refuse to listen. A microphone on a wooden table records all the noises generated from the floor up to the table top. These noises can be considerable, but are fairly well dampened by placing a towel under the microphone. Fluorescent lamps, especially older models, have small motors that hum. Most of us have learned not to hear this humming, but nevertheless a machine records it.

Any field researcher should carry a hardbacked notebook. Even if fieldnotes are recorded on the tape with the interview, or are recorded on a separate tape that contains nothing but fieldnotes, the notebook is needed to record other information and to continue the redundancy of data tracking. This other information includes directions to an informant's house, mileage, topics that should be followed up at the next interview, and names of grandchildren (drawing a family tree for each informant with names and ages is important). This is the information interviewers need with them, not on a tape that may be in the hands of a transcriptionist.

The colored pens in the camera bag are used to label on the tape and the plastic case for the tape, and write in the notebook used for fieldnotes. The colored pens allow certain kinds of information to be found at a glance (e.g., mileage is recorded in green so at the end of a week, the numbers are easily found and turned in for reimbursement). Colored pens are also useful in coding certain kinds of interactions or interviews. Interviews that are not tape-recorded for some reason, so that only fieldnotes exist, can be marked with a distinct color. Telephone contacts are recorded in a second color, and tape-recorded interviews documented in a third.

4

ETHICAL ISSUES AND ETHICAL APPROVAL

MARLENE Z. COHEN

Naturalistic researchers are very aware that ethical issues are inherent in every study. These issues begin with the identification of a problem to study—after all, we study only that which we value or deem to be important. The close relationships that hermeneutic phenomenological researchers form with their informants also increase the attention that must be given to ethical issues in research. The ethical concerns continue throughout the study and, therefore, deserve particular attention in hermeneutic phenomenological research and in a book describing phenomenological research.

The first issue likely to arise is the difference between the responsibilities of a nurse and those of a researcher. This issue is even more complex when the nurse has clinical responsibility for a particular informant.

Although some nurses have conducted research with people for whom they are providing nursing care, doing so raises many problems, and being clear to the informant about the responsibilities is critically important. When the roles of caregiver and researcher are not separate, there is always concern about how openly and honestly informants can describe experiences without fear that their care will be affected. The purpose of the research may well direct researchers to conduct research with informants to whom they are not providing nursing care.

Phenomenologists recognize the human connection that people develop as they discuss a lived experience and the responsibility this connection holds for both parties. Gurevitch (1990) presented a useful discussion of the responsibility to speak, to listen, and to respond. The researcher's dilemma is that speaking or responding too quickly with information may prevent obtaining an understanding of the other's lived experience. The responsibility of the investigator to the research needs to be balanced with the need to ensure that informants have health information they need and that they are not left distressed after talking about sensitive topics. Examples from our research, which illustrate ways to handle these issues, will be included in the following discussion.

Another important issue is the need for the researcher to have a safe place to discuss the data and research process. The stories informants share are often very difficult to hear and arouse emotions in the listener. Unless some debriefing is included, the researcher may limit the information revealed in subtle, even nonverbal ways and may fail to see important data when analysis is conducted. Finally, the researcher may simply never complete the project or fail to complete it in a timely way because of the emotions evoked. Bracketing, discussed in Chapter 1, is also important as a way of examining personal commitments and prejudices prior to beginning data collection. Bracketing helps ensure that researchers' biases are reduced in both data collection and analysis.

Inclusion of both genders and members of minority groups in research is also an ethical issue. Accurate descriptions and analysis are needed. Use of consultants or co-investigators who match the informants' life experiences, combined with sensitive interviewing and confirmation of analysis with the informants and others from the appropriate group, are useful strategies to meet these needs.

Issues that are of concern to Institutional Review Boards (IRBs) include confidentiality of data and sensitive ways to obtain informants.

The latter is particularly important when informants are sick or recruited at a time when they are vulnerable. The issue of risks versus benefits is yet another instance in which researchers need to know their audience—the IRB—and provide its members with the information they want in the way they want it.

HISTORY

A variety of important events led to the formation of IRBs to evaluate research proposals. The first of these events was the Nuremberg Tribunals, trials for Nazi war criminals. When these activities were publicized, it led to development of the Nuremberg Code in 1949. This code was for biomedical research, but it applies to research with humans in general. It included minimum standards and was developed to have standards for the trials of Nazi war criminals. The guidelines concerned voluntary consent; the option of withdrawal from studies; protection from physical and mental suffering, injury, disability, and death; and a balance of risks and benefits. The Helsinki declaration, based on the Nuremberg Code, was developed in 1964 and revised in 1975 by the World Medical Assembly. This declaration differentiated therapeutic research from nontherapeutic (in therapeutic research, the patient may benefit from the experimental treatment, whereas nontherapeutic research is done to generate knowledge to benefit future but not current patients). Nontherapeutic studies require greater care to protect those involved, and there must be strong justification to expose healthy volunteers to risks.

The Tuskegee experiment is another important event in the history of research ethics. The Tuskegee syphilis study was conducted from 1932 to 1972, a period of 40 years. The U.S. Public Health Service started this study of syphilis in black men in the small rural town of Tuskegee, Alabama, to determine the natural course of syphilis in adult black men. There were two groups, 400 untreated men and 200 controls (men without syphilis). Among the troubling aspects of this project is that the research participants were not informed of the purpose and procedure of the study. In addition, in 1936, it was clear that men with syphilis had developed complications, including blindness. In fact, 10 years later, the death rate for the infected men was twice that of the control group. By 1940, penicillin was found to be an effective treatment. Rather than offer this treatment to the men in this study, the research team continued to follow the men without treating them, and, in fact, there is evidence that the research team worked to prevent the men from receiving treatment. Professional publications about this study and its results began in 1936 and occurred every 4 to 6 years. In 1969, the study was continued by the Centers for Disease Control (CDC). The study was stopped in 1972 after a *Washington Star* account sparked public outcry about the study. It was only after this outcry that the Department of Health, Education, and Welfare stopped the study. The study was found to be "ethically unjustified," although the racial implications were addressed only much later. In 1996, President Clinton apologized to the Tuskegee survivors who were left untreated for syphilis for decades as part of this study. He said, "To our African American citizens, I am sorry that your Federal Government orchestrated a study so clearly racist" (Mitchell, 1997, p. 10).

Although issues of this kind are less likely to be problems in phenomenological research, attention must be given to ethics in all research. Despite the fact that the Nuremberg Code and Helsinki declaration were both adopted, unethical research continues. In his 1966 article, Beecher discussed 22 examples of unethical studies from published literature. The examples included lack of consent, withholding of known effective treatments, and unnecessary risks to the health and lives of subjects. Although some unethical research may result from thoughtlessness and carelessness rather than willful disregard for people, Beecher cautioned that pressures for funding, promotion, and tenure may contribute to unethical research practices. Surely, these pressures have not decreased since 1966.

Regard for people is at the heart of the philosophies that guide hermeneutic phenomenological research. There is also less distance between researchers and informants in this approach than in some others, as researchers and informants are most likely to be people sitting face to face, often in the informants' home. Because trust is vital to obtaining the data we seek, researchers need to keep the informants' vulnerability in mind and do nothing to violate their trust.

Beyond following the letter of the law, or rules, it is also important to follow the spirit of the law. This, for example, means that consent is a process, not simply a document to sign. As interviews continue over time, informants need to be clear about what they are agreeing to do;

they must know that they can withdraw their consent and decide not to participate at any point.

INSTITUTIONAL REVIEW BOARDS

IRBs are committees that review research. The first federal policy statement about protecting research subjects with an IRB review was issued in 1966. In 1974, the Department of Health, Education, and Welfare passed the National Research Act, which required that all research involving human subjects have institutional review. The Department of Health and Human Services revised these guidelines in 1981 and in 1983. These regulations call for obtaining and documenting informed consent and for establishing IRBs; they set criteria for exempt, expedited, and completely reviewed proposals. IRBs are composed of at least five members who have varied backgrounds and include nonresearchers, such as ministers, lawyers, and people not within the institution. They are charged to review research to protect the rights of subjects.

When applying for approval from an IRB, researchers need to know their audience. Boards vary in what kinds of information they need and how they work. Their task is to ensure that the research participant is protected. Some committees take that to mean that they also need to review the science of a proposal, because it would be unethical to have individuals involved in "bad science," because it would at best be wasting their time. This is an extreme position. IRBs vary in their knowledge and understanding of phenomenological research. Some preparatory discussion with members of the IRB may be helpful if they are not familiar with this methodology. Being prepared to discuss the philosophical basis and use of this method in other research may be useful. Most IRBs are concerned with protecting the health and safety of subjects, which includes mental distress. Having well-documented contingency plans for how informants could be referred in the event that they require clinical psychological intervention may be helpful.

There are three levels of review:

1. Exempt studies are those that do not require review because they are deemed to pose no known risks to patients. Phenomenological studies are often considered exempt because data are obtained in interviews.

2. Expedited studies involve minimal risk, which means risks experienced are those one might experience in daily life. The IRB chair reviews these studies.

3. Complete review by the committee is conducted for other studies when more potential risks are involved.

Individual IRBs have individual guidelines and make decisions about the level of review required for phenomenological studies. Most committees view these studies as exempt studies or at least give an expedited review. However, we have encountered committees that have decided to give these proposals full review because interviews are tape-recorded, and there may be risks to confidentiality. The level of the review is determined by the IRB and not by the individual researcher.

IRBs want information about risks and benefits. The fact that nurses who do phenomenological research are skilled interviewers is a clear benefit. Patients often comment that it is helpful to them to talk with someone about experiences that they often have never talked about before. At the very least, informants are contributing to research in nursing aimed at improving care and may well see this as a benefit. The most serious risk is that people are talking about important, often emotionally charged events, and this may result in their feeling distress. Although this is not a serious risk, because people reveal what they want to reveal, it is always wise to be able to make mental health referrals, should these seem necessary. Having this support available may also be important to the researcher, as will be discussed below.

ANONYMITY AND CONFIDENTIALITY

A common part of the ethical agreement made between researchers and informants is that the data will be published or presented in a way that preserves informants' anonymity and confidentiality. This is sometimes difficult to accomplish when the demands of confidentiality are balanced with the need to present detailed information about the informants. This detail is an important context for the findings. I have often discussed with informants plans for disguising them. In one study, the pseudonym I selected for an informant happened to be her maiden name. In another study, a nurse informant talked about her husband's death. Because many of the nurses she worked with knew about this experience, and because it was a sensitive topic, I asked her to read what I planned to publish about this experience. I told her it was a wonderful example but that if she had any concerns about it being published, or the way it was written, I would be happy to make whatever changes she suggested. She was comfortable with what was written. However, I have had other informants ask me to delete details of their experiences for fear that they will be recognized. These wishes need to be honored.

GENDER AND MINORITY INCLUSION

Giving voice to those who need to be heard is an important aspect of phenomenological research and can be extended to the inclusion of members of minority groups. African Americans are likely to know about the Tuskegee experiment. If they do not know about it, they at least are likely to have experienced racism in our society, if not in our health care environments. Special efforts are needed to recruit minorities.

In addition, incentives may be important in recruiting minorities. Wineman and Durand (1992) distinguished between *incentives*, clearly stated up front and given to prompt someone to action, and *rewards*, which are given after the fact to recognize some service or achievement and are often not stated up front. Although there is controversy in the literature about the use of monetary incentives, because they may be coercive when the amount is large or the person offered the incentive is poor, providing money as an incentive may be useful to consider.

In two projects (Phillips & Cohen, 1998; Phillips, Cohen, & Moses, 1999), it became clear that there was a need to pay some African Americans a small amount of money ($25) as appreciation for participating. Although some women were willing to participate without this compensation, there was a need to recruit low-income women, and for this group, the money was important.

RESEARCHER DEBRIEFING

This is another example of when a research team is like a good marriage. It is important to have a partner whom you can trust completely to listen as you share difficult things you have heard and to validate that you have done all you need to do. An example of this is in research conducted by Phillips and Cohen (1998). One woman told Phillips that an abnormality had been found on her mammogram. Phillips talked with her about the biopsy both before and after it was done. Fortunately, the biopsy showed the mass was not malignant. However, the conversations with the informant were difficult, and it helped Phillips to have a colleague with whom to talk about this.

Ethical issues are inherent in all research and it is important to attend to them. This chapter has discussed the evolution of IRBs and key issues to which they and hermeneutic phenomenological researchers need to attend.

5

SAMPLING

RICHARD H. STEEVES

Sampling in hermeneutic phenomenological research means about the same as it does in other research, even though it is approached very differently. Sampling implies that a researcher is choosing informants because those informants might have something to say about an experience they share with others. Hermeneutic phenomenological researchers, as stated in Chapter 1, are interested in how individuals express the language of their tradition and how the language of a tradition is expressed through the individual (Gadamer, 1989; Kockelmans, 1975).

The method of choosing a sample that will allow access to the individual and the tradition or language is different in hermeneutic phenomenological research than in other approaches. Also, the approach to sampling in hermeneutic phenomenological research varies depending on the question being asked or the particular phenomenon of interest. There are numerous ways of organizing a discussion of sampling; one way is to consider the phenomenon of interest in one of three frames: the experiences of place, the experiences of events in time, and ways of talking about experiences. The division is, of necessity, artificial. Most hermeneutic phenomenological researchers are interested in all three at the same time and would say that no single phenomenon can be understood in isolation. For instance, a place cannot be understood separately from the events that occur in the place or the manners of talking of the people who frequent the place. But it is heuristically useful to consider these categories separately. It is important to keep in mind that hermeneutic phenomenological research is aimed at understanding the way people interpret their world. This way of framing the discussion of sampling is inspired by Merleau-Ponty's (1962) seminal work, *Phenomenology of Perception,* and the work of Gadamer (1989). Merleau-Ponty argues that people are first and foremost a body in space. More than that, being in a specific place is always a part of every experience. He also argues that events, or time, is essential to experience: "I am myself time" (p. 421), he says, and "Subjectivity [experience] is not in time because it takes up or lives time and merges with the cohesion of a life" (p. 422). Gadamer (1989) is interested in interpretation or hermeneutics and how people make sense of their experiences. His concern is the way people use language to tell themselves and others about their experiences. Thus, it seems appropriate for a hermeneutic phenomenological researcher to use the heuristic of organizing a discussion into the three frames, experiencing place, experiencing events over time, and ways of talking about experiences.

EXPERIENCING PLACE

Anthropologists have been studying places for a long time. But anthropologists are usually interested in places because culture is acted out in those places. A number of anthropologists, including Geertz (1973), call what they do when they study culture hermeneutics. That is because they have the same larger goal as hermeneutic phenomenological researchers—understanding how people interpret their world—even if they ask dif-

ferent kinds of questions (see Chapter 1). For the hermeneutic phenomenological researcher, it is useful to look at places and how the experience of place is a part of the phenomenon in which we are interested.

As I have stated above, when I studied bone marrow transplantation, I
was interested in the inpatient unit where the transplantation took place
because this is where patients suffered the worst complications. I wanted
to learn how these patients and their families interpreted the suffering
they were experiencing. I was interested in a great deal more than just
the place, naturally, but I will confine my discussion to how I learned
about the informant's interpretation of or experience of place.

The world of bone marrow transplant patients appeared to consist of
ever-tightening concentric circles. These patients moved to a large West
Coast city for their transplant and, at first, had access to the entire city
and environs. But as their "conditioning" for the transplant began in the
outpatient clinic, they were confined to that clinic and the neighborhood that surrounded the clinic and hospital. This area of the city was
called "pill hill" because of all the clinics and hospitals. Eventually, as the
conditioning progressed, patients were admitted to the hospital, and
their world shrank again. When they were experiencing the most difficult part of the bone marrow transplant, they were confined to their
room, and many were confined to a corner of their rooms completely
sealed off with plastic curtains to prevent them from coming in contact
with pathogens.

My major interest was the inpatient unit, because this is where patients and families spent most or their time. The unit consisted of 10 patient rooms and the various support rooms common to inpatient floors.
The bone marrow transplant patients were required to live there for
weeks, perhaps months at a time. The inpatient unit became their new
home. News from the far-off cities they called home was important but
seemed tantalizingly distant and unreal. What happened in the unit was
immediate and important. Even while they were confined to a single
corner of their room, they were interested in how the other patients on
the unit were doing: who was surviving, who was dying. The nurses con-
sciously tried to keep news of other patients from spreading and even
evaded direct questions, but the patients and their families always found
out.

I wanted to find out as much as I could about this place as the patients
and their families experienced it. But how does a researcher sample to

learn about a place? The obvious answer is by being there. Lincoln and Guba (1985) and numerous others have referred to this kind of data collection as using the researcher, or the self, as instrument. Because this term has become a regular part of the lexicon of qualitative researchers, it requires some attention. The idea of using the self as instrument is fraught with difficulties. The notion is alienating and unworkable in that it asks a researcher to treat him- or herself as object rather than subject. We are first and foremost subjects to ourselves, and it takes a wrenching and radical reduction of our consciousness to treat ourselves as objects. One could, of course, argue that Western culture has created numerous situations that call for just such a wrenching. Thinking of ourselves as objects makes it too easy to deny that we are interacting, interpreting, and creating meaning in everything we experience. Second, treating oneself as an instrument, as an inanimate, adjustable piece of equipment, offers a sense of the mechanical to the process of interpretation that is unfortunate. I am not arguing a naive naturalism. It is just that in our present technological state, the machines we create function very differently from their makers (Dreyfus, 1979). Machines and people are not much alike. Thus, the notion of the researcher as instrument is inaccurate and can be misleading. It may be more useful to talk about the researcher taking the place of the instrument.

As an observer, I watched and took notes about the unit: what it looked like, what it smelled like, what it sounded like. It was important to sample over time. The unit was not the same place at 3 in the morning as it was at 9 in the morning when fellows, residents, and attending physicians made their rounds. Sunday afternoons were different from Tuesday afternoons, when all the specialists—radiation, physical therapy, and psychiatry—came to see the patients . The bone marrow transplant unit was different the week of the 4th of July, when I began my study, than it was the week of Christmas, when I ended it. Seasons change the way people experience their world. A secular and political holiday celebrated with fireworks creates a different atmosphere from the formal reverence of a high religious holiday. The unit was more than atmosphere and rooms and halls; it was a social world as well. I learned that this social world was important to patients and families as they interpreted their experiences.

By being present, I learned a great deal about the bone marrow transplant unit. Generally, I was treated like a friend of the family of the men in my study. I was already interviewing patients and families and was finding out about their social life in the unit. I did not interview staff members and unit workers. But I listened as they interacted with patients and families, and I talked with staff as family would talk with the staff.

Had the staff been the major thrust of my research, as it was with Mannon (1985) in his study of a burn unit, I would have done as he did and talked with social workers, chaplains, and radiation technologists. I would also have studied the physicians: residents, attending physicians, and fellows. But these people were not generally a large part of the everyday world of the patients and families. From the patient and family point of view, the unit was peopled by the nursing staff and the housekeeping staff. The physicians were important, naturally, because of the decisions they made, and the rituals of medicine, such as rounds, affected some of the life of the unit every morning. For the largest part of the day, however, physicians were not present on the unit. My observations had also made it clear that the life on the unit was different at night than it was during the day, different on weekends than it was during the week. Not many staff members rotated shifts, and the weekends were generally staffed by people who chose to work then for whatever reasons.

I stayed with the patients and families and talked with the people who came in contact with them. I tried to learn about the place as the patients and families did. I learned who among the nurses were "hard core" and forced patients to exercise and perform hygiene tasks when they were exhausted and wanted to beg off. I learned who on the housekeeping staff was willing to run an errand or sit and gossip for awhile. I learned who family and patients used to gain information or intervene in protocols for them. In short, I leaned how the social world of the unit became a part of how patients and families interpreted their experiences.

EXPERIENCING EVENTS OVER TIME

Events are experienced as occurrences, happenings, or things that "take place." But events do not take place as much as they take time in a place. How people experience these events over time is of considerable interest to hermeneutic phenomenological researchers. In the study I conducted with caregivers of people with cancer (Steeves, 1996), I used a hospice to recruit my informants. Because I was interested in the experiences of people caring for dying patients, I recruited family caregivers of patients who were at home rather than those in the residential or inpatient part of hospice, who were being cared for by professionals.

Random sampling is not in keeping with the hermeneutic phenomenological method. Choosing people to talk to by picking their names from a hat is no basis for a relationship at all and, therefore, not a reliable method of gaining in-depth information. I did what is usually referred to as purposive sampling. I wanted a sample of people who were being forced to make sense out of caring for a dying family member.

I did not have a large pool of potential informants. The number of available informants who met the criteria for the study did not exceed by much the number I could recruit and interview, given the time and resources I had. That is, most of the time, I tried to recruit all who were available. At times, my schedule became so full that I could not interview a potential informant, but there were also weeks that went by during which I was ready but could not find a new informant.

One of the tenets of hermeneutic phenomenological research is to see informants not in terms of groups of individual characteristics that can be seen as variables but as people who offer a picture of what it is like to be themselves as they make sense of an important experience. Therefore, a hermeneutic phenomenological researcher does not usually set out to have as many elderly informants as younger ones, as many males as females, as many of one race as another. There are times when these differences are salient. But care should be taken that picking out characteristics such as these to guide sampling does not oversimplify the complex human world that affects the way people interpret their experiences.

Some of the informants in my study were better with language than others, some were more introspective than others, and some simply liked me better than others and therefore were willing to tell me more. Although the stories of all informants are valuable, not all informants are alike. Some stories are more detailed than others, and it is easier for some informants to tell stories than it is for others. Eliciting the story of each informant is not always easy, but it is the researcher's responsibility.

In the caregiver study, I used a two-tier system of sampling. Since then, I have regularly employed variations of this system. The protocol I developed called for two interviews with the caregivers before the death of the patient: one shortly after admission to hospice and a second in 3 weeks. A third interview, 6 weeks after the death, was the final one. But my protocol also called for following a small number of informants, the second tier, more intensively.

My coinvestigator, Marilyn King, followed one woman, and I followed two men and a woman. With this second tier of informants, we averaged six interviews instead of the three planned. We went to the hospital with informants, attended church, were guests at their parties, and talked to them regularly on the telephone. We chose this second tier of informants because, as they began to tell us about how they understood their worlds, we found in their texts themes and refrains that had appeared in a number of the interviews with other informants. In some small part, their ability to express that tradition out of which they were interpreting the world played a part in choosing them as exemplars. A text has to be rich and thick for numerous themes and strains to become apparent so that they can be compared to other texts.

In the bereavement study, I also used a two-tier system of sampling. I followed 18 widows and widowers over a period of as close to 2 years as I could manage, given my resources. All of these informants were subject to the same intense data collection as the small sample in the caregiver study. But I also wanted some of the advantage that comes with having a larger sample, specifically, a better knowledge of the variety of ways to live through and interpret bereavement. I talked with hospice nurses and social workers and asked them to help me choose a second sample. I asked them to identify people who were going through bereavement in a unique way, in a way that was surprising. I was asking hospice people to provide me with clues to variety.

This approach of having hospice workers tell me of informants I should recruit offered both advantages and dangers. The advantage, of course, was that I knew something about the informant and could decide whether interviewing that person would add to the variety of the data. Hospice workers generally listen carefully to patients and family members and are often very sensitive to what is going on in a household. The disadvantage was that I could be merely sampling the prejudices of the hospice workers. This is a danger any time a researcher asks someone else to recommend informants in a study. For instance, if a hospice worker has an idea about the orthodox way to grieve, any deviation from that might be considered unusual grieving for that worker. This is a problem when the hospice worker's notion of orthodoxy is unusual, and he or she categorizes as unusual what would be considered normal by a wider society. The opposite, identifying the unusual as the ordinary is also a problem. One approach to alleviating this problem is checking information on an offered informant with another member of the hospice staff. Of course, this does not address the problem of an institutionally shared unique perspective. But one hopes for the best.

WAYS OF TALKING ABOUT EXPERIENCE

As was pointed out above, hermeneutic phenomenological social scientists are interested in both the tradition from which an individual approaches interpreting experience and the specific way the individual expresses that tradition. According to Gadamer (1989) and Kockelmans (1975), the tradition is language, the way people talk to themselves and others as they interpret their world. A problem lies in identifying the tradition or the shared language that makes up a tradition.

Considering everyone who speaks English to have come from the same tradition is not very useful. The notion of a tradition or a perspective toward interpreting experience must be more finely drawn than that. Let us take, for instance, my own neighborhood. One family down the street is Sufi, another family is born-again Christian, and a third is Sunni Muslim, second-generation immigrants from Iran. In all the families, English is the first language. But if I were to interview each of the families and ask them to explain how they interpret grief and bereavement, I am quite sure that I would find they were using different traditions as they interpreted events. Just as sharing a neighborhood and a primary language does not mean sharing an interpretation of grief, sharing ethnicity, race, age, religion, or socioeconomic status does not guarantee a shared tradition, either. In fact, people usually share the tradition out of which they interpret some events with one group and a different tradition with another. For instance, when George Will, the columnist, writes about baseball, I read him with enthusiasm; when he writes about politics, I avoid his work. He and I share some traditions but not others.

Those people who share a tradition or a way of talking about experiences are people who share a specialized knowledge about a set of rules and options that govern how they can talk in specific social situations

(Garfinkel, 1972; Gumperz & Hymes, 1972). That is, although I might be able to learn the rules of a particular way of talking about experiences and might even learn to understand what is being said and why, I would not really be able to generate the kind of talk that would make me a real member of the group that talks that way. For example, it might be argued that since millions of Americans listen to Tom Brokaw every night and understand what he says, we must share the same way of talking about things. However, television and movies are not interactive. I merely listen to TV. I do not have to respond, and response is necessary to master a language. Few of the people who listen to *NBC Nightly News* can generate the speech that would put them in the same tradition of interpreting as the broadcasters.

In the bereavement study, I interviewed a man named Wilford Nelson (I have changed all the names in this text) whose wife was dying of metastatic cancer. Then, I was given the opportunity to recruit Mimi Nelson into the study. She was from the same county and was losing her husband to lung cancer. I relished the opportunity because I thought I would be able to have a second view of the same group of people going through a similar loss. I was wrong.

My assumption was that since they lived in the same rural county and had the same last name, they would be kin and be part of the same tradition or way of talking about experience. These two families are indeed kin, Mimi having married into the Nelson family. But the kinship tie between Mimi's side of the family and Wilford's is so far in the past that neither group remembers exactly how they are linked. When asked by outsiders, they usually find it easier to say that they coincidentally have the same last name and are not kin. Wilford owns a section of land, 640 acres, and his two brothers each own at least twice that much. The land in this county is not particularly good; the topsoil is less than 2 inches deep in most places. Logging and grazing cattle are the only sources of income in the county, outside of guard work at the maximum-security prison.

On the other hand, Mimi's husband owns a doublewide trailer on a piece of land just big enough for the trailer and a little garden. Mimi's husband works for Wilford's family off and on when there is logging to do or hay to cut. They do not attend the same church, although they are all Baptist. Members of the two families do not talk with each other on any regular basis.

When Wilford was taking care of his wife, he often would bypass the hospice nurse when he had a question and call his physician directly. This physician knew Wilford and his family socially and made a number of house calls. Wilford knew how to navigate the health care system and eventually had at his disposal respiratory therapists, physical therapists, home health aides, chaplains, and nurses.

Mimi rarely talked to the doctor who was caring for her husband. She took pride in the fact that she and her family could take care of her husband. They did not want any outsiders involved except for the nurse, whom they grew to know and like. While her husband was undergoing chemotherapy and radiation, Mimi continued to treat him at home. A cousin who had lost a husband to congestive heart failure told Mimi that she had seen an article in a magazine about the benefits of raisins soaked in vinegar and raisins soaked in gin for restoring health and relieving all kinds of symptoms. Mimi had both in her refrigerator and relied on the raisins when the morphine and the oxygen did not help her husband.

Whom one talks to about illness is important. Whom a patient or family member talks with can make a difference in a number of ways, including what we call compliance (i.e., doing what you are told). Wilford, to some extent, shared the doctor's way of talking about his wife's illness and its treatment and learned how to avail himself of all the benefits traditional health care has to offer. Mimi had a way of talking about illness and availed herself of different interventions.

The importance of this discussion of ways of talking about experience is not to insist that a hermeneutic phenomenological researcher talk to all the members of an informant's shared tradition to understand how a person understands an experience. The goal is to understand the individual and the tradition. The informant is being interviewed to understand the tradition or way of talking about experience, and an understanding of the tradition is necessary for understanding the individual's interpretation of the world. The way people talk about a certain topic, death and grieving or caring for the ill, for example, is the source of and the repository of interpretations of the world. The individual uses these interpretations in a unique way to understand his or her experience.

Exploring who shares a way of talking about a particular experience cannot be determined before the researcher enters the field. Funding agencies often ask or even require that women and minorities be included in samples and that recruitment procedures for these groups be specified. I am not arguing against that practice. Years of neglect and prejudice need to be remedied. Including African Americans, however, in a sample does not ensure that one will be tapping into a group of people who have the same tradition. Ethnicity and sharing a way of talking about a particular experience are not the same thing. Even what seems obvious—that an immediate family living together would share a way of talking about experiences—is not necessarily true. If interpretations in a family were homogenous, perhaps, marriages would not break up.

Determining who shares a way of talking about experiences is problematic and can be determined only through careful data collection. Groups of people who talk about a few topics, a few experiences, to each other in the same way do not correspond to demographic markers and cannot be identified in advance of fieldwork.

GUESSING IN ADVANCE

Sampling places, experiences, and speech communities is what a hermeneutic phenomenological researcher does. Funding agencies and dissertation committees need to know how the sampling is going to be carried out in the field; in addition, they usually want to know what the sample size will be. This request is not at odds with the philosophical underpinnings of the hermeneutic phenomenological method. Of course, there is considerable information that can be gained only from being in the field, observing, and interviewing for some time, but that should not prevent one from being accountable in advance for time spent.

The estimation of time to be spent or the amount of contact needed with informants and the number of informants needed is not as easy as calculating power in statistics. Ideally, a researcher would have the freedom and the resources to continue to collect data until nothing new was being observed or recorded, no matter how long that takes. But this is usually not the case, and the hermeneutic phenomenological researcher must rely on previous studies and clinical experience.

In the bone marrow transplant study, the time frame for each informant was determined by the clinical protocol. The protocol for patients started on the first day of transplantation and was complete 100 days later, if the patient lived that long. My difficulty in that study was determining the number of informants to follow. I wanted to follow at least five because statistically 66% would die during the process and I wanted to have more than one informant left to talk about what it was like to survive. Interviewing at least five would not ensure that I would have a survivor in my sample, but it would increase my chances. I wanted to follow fewer than 10 because I wanted to follow each informant intensely rather than spread my attention over a larger group. I completed the study with a sample of six informants.

The caregiver study offered other problems. A review of the literature on caregivers of dying patients led me to believe that the experience was not as intense and variable day to day as having a bone marrow transplant. Thus, I believed I could use a larger sample, 30 at least. My own clinical experience in hospice and the advice of other hospice nurses led me to plan on collecting data at three different points: (a) when a patient was first admitted to hospice; (b) a few weeks later, when a rapid decline in health was typical; and (c) a few weeks after the death, when informants might be ready to look back on the experience as a whole.

I returned to a smaller sample in the bereavement study. The literature on the process and progress of bereavement in the elderly is equivocal. That is, there is little agreement on what happens for an elderly person after the loss of a spouse. I became convinced that close attention needed to be paid to the day-to-day experiences of these people, and that meant a smaller sample followed more closely. Also, the literature suggested that anywhere from 6 months to 2 years was the length of bereavement; therefore, I needed to follow my sample for an extended period of time (see Steeves & Kahn, 1999).

Of course, a number of practical considerations also play into estimates of sample size, such as expectations of dissertation committee members, availability of funds, extent of teaching loads for faculty, and the like. But these considerations affect all researchers and do not affect the work of hermeneutic phenomenological researchers more or less heavily than others. The scientifically important criterion for determining sample size for the hermeneutic phenomenological researcher is the intensity of the contact needed to gather sufficient data regarding a phenomenon or experience. This intensity is measured in both length of time it takes for an event to occur, for example, 100 days or 2 years, and how often a participant should be contacted to understand the changes undergone, for example, daily or once every few weeks. As the intensity of contact increases, in terms of both length of time and frequency of contact, the size of the sample will necessarily decrease. An estimate of the amount of intensity needed should be based on a review of extant studies and clinical experience.

6

HOW TO CONDUCT RESEARCH

Dᴀᴠɪᴅ L. Kᴀʜɴ

In this chapter, I will discuss how to collect data using the hermeneutic phenomenological approach. First, I will offer and elaborate on the metaphor of building a field text through data collection as a useful way for the beginner to think about how to conduct research. I will then discuss interviews, fieldnotes, and the collection of other documents, all of which can be thought of as layers of the field text. Finally, I will end with some basic advice for new researchers about building data collection skills.

Life is experienced in the present at hand but not studied, analyzed, or interpreted in that same moment. Experience, and the meanings that arise through experience, can be studied only in the past, after the fact, so to speak, or after the experience has been lived. Thus, whether I take a retrospective approach in a study, such as asking African American women to describe the illness they experience from heart disease, or a prospective approach to a phenomenon, such as following hospice patients dying of cancer, my concern is with fixing or situating the experiences of my informants and myself in some form that will allow me to consider it later, to consult it again, and to return to it as necessary.

Situating the experience of informants, for the most part, involves language or textual data. Informants tell or inform (hence that label) about their experience in words. Observations are also inscribed in words, written down in some way. Thus, the metaphor of a text, which is created through data collection and can be read in data analysis, is a useful way to think about the process of this method.

Data collection, then, involves the construction of a multilayered text about "the meaning of the human experiences under inquiry" (Steeves & Kahn, 1995, p. 186). For example, in my nursing home study (Kahn, 1990), one layer of the text was constructed from interviews with the elderly residents in the privacy of their rooms. These interviews were audiotape-recorded and transcribed. Other conversations took place as I participated in social interactions typical of life in this nursing home. Whether these interactions were structured, such as attending the daily exercise classes for residents, or unstructured, such as joining in the conversation of a small group of residents sitting in the nursing home lobby, I described them in detail in notes made as soon as possible after the interaction occurred. Traditionally called fieldnotes, these written accounts of observing and participating in social interaction added another layer to the field text.

Written descriptions of things that are observed, such as details of the environments in which the experiences being studied take place, often constitute a layer of the field text. In the nursing home study, for example, fieldnotes that described the level of noise, the different patterns of staff activity, and the way residents decorated their rooms became important components of an analytic theme involving a dialectic between the nursing home as institution and as home (Kahn, 1999).

Often, documents collected in the field may add yet another layer to the text. It is difficult to predict in advance what documents will be included, as this varies widely from study to study. Some documents, such as newsletters from the nursing home mentioned above, may be sought out by the investigator. Some documents may be surprises, such as writings offered spontaneously by informants in the study to illustrate symbolic aspects of their own experience.

Thus, the field text constructed in data collection is not only multilayered, but also symbolic and distanced from the experiences of interest in order to allow hermeneutic interpretation (Ricoeur, 1981), which forms the basis of data analysis in the hermeneutic phenomenological method. That the text is distanced from the experience enables objectification and hence interpretation (Gallagher, 1992; Ricoeur, 1981)—the metaphor that fits is that of a person stepping back from a painting to better view it as a whole.

INTERVIEWS AND INTERVIEWING

Interviews are an essential piece of data collection in most qualitative methods of inquiry. Consequently, there is an abundance of literature that deals with interviews and techniques of interviewing in considerable depth. Students and researchers new to qualitative inquiry have a wide variety of options to choose from in reading about interviews and interviewing technique. In my own development as an interviewer, I found discussions of interviewing by Spradley (1979) from an ethnographic perspective and by Taylor and Bogdan (1984) from the perspective of symbolic interactionism to be particularly clear and practical, and I have used their ideas in the development of the hermeneutic phenomenological method. More recent discussions of interviewing that are consistent with my own ideas include Denzin (1989), Holstein and Gubrium (1995), Yow (1994), and Fontana and Frey (1994). Although various methods may differ in the philosophical assumptions about inquiry and in the theoretical perspective in which phenomena under study are viewed, the basic elements of interviewing technique and the methodological issues that need to be considered are similar across methods.

A basic premise of the hermeneutic phenomenological method is that a driving force of human consciousness is to make sense of experience. In general, people try to reach this understanding by interpreting their lives as they occur by treating them as narratives that are unfolding. In other words, the understanding people have of their world and life situation and the meaning they have made of this is usually contained in the narratives or stories they tell, first to themselves to make sense of their own experience; then to family, friends, and other social actors in their lives; and finally to any social scientists who come asking (Benner & Wrubel, 1989; Dreyfus, 1991; Geertz, 1973; Sandelowski, 1993; SmithBattle, 1994; Steeves & Kahn, 1995). As Denzin (1989) argued, these narratives are always intensely autobiographical and inherently meaningful, and hence the natural focus of inquiry is aimed at understanding the meaning of human experience.

Interviews can elicit a variety of types of data through the kinds of questions that are asked. As Steeves (1992b) noted, these types of data include the specifics of word use, as illustrated by a study that asked informants to describe what came to mind when the word *hopefulness* was mentioned (Hinds & Martin, 1988), as well as explanations, as illustrated in studies that ask informants to explain the decisions they made when confronted, for example, with a particular diagnosis or a variety of treatment options. Another type of data that can be elicited from interviews is narrative data. Obviously, it is this type of data that is of most interest to us who use the hermeneutic phenomenological method.

An example of the richness of narrative data can be seen in the following excerpt of an interview I conducted with an 89-year-old woman who lived in a nursing home. When asked early in the interview to talk about changes she had experienced due to old age, the informant first offered up the following explanation, assuming that an explanation was what I wanted:

> It is very hard to explain to someone who hasn't done it. You know, it is different than I expected . . . all the things that happen to you that you never really thought about when you were young. Sometimes I think I should write a book but what would I say. You have to be old to know what it is like, I guess.

I then indicated my interest in her specific stories about things that happened to her in old age by asking, "Can you tell me about some of the things that happened to you?" This kind of query is an example of what Holstein and Gubrium (1995) technically conceptualized as *activating narrative construction* by indicating your openness to a narrative response and orienting the subsequent conversation to a narrative focus (p. 39). The informant responded with a story about the losses she had experienced in recent years; the story captures poignantly an aspect of the meaning old age had for her, based on her life experience:

I had brothers I grew up with, let's see, nine brothers. They respected me and [were] very kind. I couldn't have one brother come and see me [without] another brother would come and see me. Always coming to see me. Now they're gone, all those boys. Little by little, little by little. Little by little they died. [A brief account of each brother's death then follows.] I also had very good friends. They too have got old. And they're gone.

In the hermeneutic phenomenological method, to elicit narrative data I aim for interviews that resemble conversations. This differs from interviews that are tightly structured and use a more directive style, such as interviews with guides that specify questions that must be asked, a specific wording for each question, and an order of asking. Our interviews are akin to what Morse (1991) described as *interactive interviews* and Holstein and Gubrium (1995) described as an *active interview*. In this kind of interview, information is exchanged between informant and interviewer in both directions, the format is relatively unstructured, and the emphasis of the interviewer is on listening to whatever the informant says as opposed to guiding and controlling the conversation.

The questions asked of the informant are not the same as the analytic questions asked of the data (Steeves, Kahn, & Cohen, 1996). It is the job of the researcher to answer questions of scientific interest and construct explanations and theories. For example, in the present study of hospice cancer patients by Kahn and Steeves, the informants are asked not to explain what a good death is for them but instead to relate their experiences in detail. When informants are asked an analytic question, such as defining a good death, they may not necessarily confine their responses to their own experience but may draw on religious dogma, popular psychology, or other sources and end up explaining what they believe they believe about a good death. The hermeneutic phenomenological tradition holds that informants have already interpreted the meaning of their lives (including the process of dying) in the very act of turning their experiences into stories or narrative texts that can be told.

There are two basic ways to solicit these narratives in the context of a conversation. The difference is based on where the informant is in relation to the experience that you will talk about—either the experience is primarily in the past (the experience of being treated for breast cancer or the experience of childbirth, for example) or the experience is ongoing (the experience of being a cancer patient in hospice or the experience of raising a child). This distinction is not completely clear-cut but should be reflected in the stance informants take and in the way they talk about the experience, that is, mostly in the past or in the present tense.

When I study informants undergoing an experience, I use a longitudinal, prospective approach. When my inquiry is focused on what has already occurred, even though to an extent it remains ongoing, I use a retrospective approach. Each approach solicits narratives in a different way.

The way to solicit narratives of experience in the prospective approach is to elicit as much detail as possible about the informant's daily life. A specific technique that has been useful for me in the past takes the form of three statements. The first statement is "tell me the most important thing that has happened to you recently" (i.e., since I was last here, since you entered the hospice program, since your husband died, since you were diagnosed with cancer—all of which arise from the phenomenon of interest in the particular study). The second statement is aimed at broadening the scope of the interview by asking the informant to tell of an important event that has the opposite emotional valance of the first narrative: "Tell me of a time recently that was particularly happy" (or difficult, depending on what the first narrative was like). The third statement is aimed at filling in as much detail about daily life as possible. It is used to establish that the interviewer is interested in the everyday aspect of living with a terminal illness, taking care of a dying person, or again experiencing whatever the phenomenon of interest is in the study. Thus, the third statement we use is: "Pick a normal day for you and tell me what happened."

The fear in letting informants direct the interview and tell their own narratives is that they will not talk about what is of interest to the researcher. If a topic is not of enough interest to the informants to be included in their narratives, however, it probably is not an important part of their experience and not worth the researcher's pursuit. It should be noted that this approach differs from traditional phenomenology, which uses a broad opening question that focuses on the phenomenon under study.

Repeated interviews over time with most informants in a study are an essential feature of the hermeneutic phenomenological method when used with a prospective approach. Repeated encounters are important in developing trust and rapport (Taylor & Bogdan, 1984). In my experience, the use of the three questions outlined above is rarely needed after rapport is developed with an informant. After a relationship has been established, most informants look forward to the opportunity of telling their story and need no prompting. Indeed, at this point, most informants begin telling additional stories of their life that help greatly in analysis by adding autobiographical context to their recent experiences. The issues of trust and rapport are discussed in more depth in Spradley (1979) and Yow (1994), among others.

When a retrospective approach in the hermeneutic phenomenological method is used, soliciting narratives of experience depends on developing interview questions that turn the informants to the experience and ask them to talk about it. This is the common approach used in many traditional phenomenological studies. An experience is identified and informants who have had and reflected on the experience are recruited. The interviews with informants begin with a general question such as, "What does this [experience] mean to you?" or "What is it like to have [this experience]?" Initial answers are then probed until the experience is fully described (Ray, 1994). Pilot interviews can be used to develop probes. This is useful for students and other novice researchers, who, I have found, are often worried about how to maintain a conversational interview with a participant. It is important, however, not to let the probes become directive or structure the interview in a predetermined way. Consistent with the preceding discussion, the probes used in these interviews would focus on eliciting narrative data as opposed to explanations or opinions.

When asking a person to turn to the experience, it is important to remain close to a level of experience that is common to everyday life. That is, it is not productive to ask participants to talk about something that from their perspective is an abstraction. Students are often interested in constructs such as health, health promotion, and quality of life. Such constructs, although meaningful to researchers participating in a disciplinary discourse of theory and research, are not particularly meaningful for other people. Asking people how they experience their health is too removed from everyday life experience. A more concrete, specific experience, however, can often be identified that would advance the discourse around the more abstract construct. For example, a student of mine, interested in health promotion and adaptation to stress in women, identified exercise as a specific experience related to this larger area. Exercise was an everyday life experience her participants were ready and able to turn to and talk about with her (Kneipp, 1993).

Sometimes, it is simply a matter of translating professional jargon. For example, Yang (1999) was interested in the effects of infertility on the marital relationship; she posed the question to the women in her study as "What is it like for you not to be able to have children" and probed for additional description that included experiences with their husbands.

Although repeated interviews over time are not necessary in a retrospective approach to the study of lived experience, I have found it useful to have at least two interviews with each informant. The second interview can be an occasion for the researcher to review the transcript of the first interview and/or the tentative findings of the study, formulated as themes, with the informant. Not only does this review help to reduce researcher bias, but it also serves as a conversation in which the informant can offer more narratives and more description of the experience under inquiry. Informants often reflect on their experience after being interviewed the first time, which leads to enriched data in the second interview.

PARTICIPATION AND OBSERVATION

Some qualitative methods such as ethnography subsume interviewing under the larger rubric of participant observation. In other methods, distinctions between participant observation and observation are important. In the hermeneutic phenomenological method, participation and observation are considered two abstract poles of a more pragmatic continuum. It is impossible to imagine observation of the social world without the possibility of social interaction or participation being inherent in that observation. And the perspective of inquiry into a particular research problem similarly precludes the researcher's total immersion without observation in the social worlds of informants. Thus, there are pragmatic distinctions I make about observations of my own participation in social interaction and observations of the places or social setting important to the inquiry at hand. What is most important is that these observations are necessary to construct a field text, providing important context and source of insight for the narrative data collected through interviews. These observations are fixed or inscribed through the technique of writing fieldnotes.

The fieldnotes I have recorded in different studies have served a number of purposes. First of all, fieldnotes have enabled me to reconstruct the physical environments or settings in which study informants spend time. For example, extensive fieldnotes I recorded in the nursing home study regarding the ambience of the nursing home were important in understanding important aspects of the experience of living in a nursing home, including the ambiguity of the environment. Careful documentation of aspects of this nursing home in terms of cleanliness, organization, and quality of care also allowed me to understand my informants' experience of "going downhill" as they understood it in terms of their physical and social decline, rather than as a problem that could be fixed by intervening in the way care was delivered. At the very least, careful descriptions of the physical settings in my fieldnotes enable me to convey such descriptions to readers later, as needed.

Similarly, in this method, fieldnotes are used to record those aspects of the interview that cannot be discerned from the transcript of the tape recording: body language, tone of voice, environmental distractions, the dress and demeanor of the informant, and the important symbols that are hanging on the walls or standing on tables and bookshelves. For example, one of the informants in Steeves's caregiver study decorated her house with stylized images of Native Americans in empty, open settings. The dominant theme in her interviews was her self-expectation that she must be courageous and silent in the face of suffering, the image she held of Native Americans.

Fieldnotes are also important in recording details that emerge or become clear after the tape recorder was turned off or is not available. In my study of frail African American elders, one informant stopped by my house and explained about a phone call she had just received from a hospital in a town more than a thousand miles away. The hospital had called her about a nephew she had not seen in 40 years. The nephew was dying of cancer, and her husband and she were in the process of preparing to leave within an hour for the long and unplanned drive to see him. This story was important in understanding her experience of family ties, and there was no time or opportunity for me to tape-record it.

Another purpose of fieldnotes in the hermeneutic phenomenological method is to provide an opportunity for reflection and self-evaluation. As a relationship evolves with an informant, deciding the best way to interact with that informant should be a conscious and deliberate process based on observations from each contact. The evaluative assessment of iterations and interview techniques in fieldnotes is important in continuing the construction of the field text and in interpretation of that text.

Finally, fieldnotes should be used to record substantive and theoretical hunches, ideas, insights, and observations. Early impressions regarding what is happening in the informant's life in terms of the goals of the research are invaluable aids in analysis, as they fix in writing the researcher's emerging understanding of the situation. At the same time, careful recording of what is initially confusing and difficult to understand is also important and often serves as clues to aspects of the informant's experience that are important to understand. This kind of note may direct more focused observations as the study proceeds.

As will be discussed in a later chapter, data analysis begins as soon as data are collected. As analysis proceeds, observations and hence fieldnotes will become more focused and specific. The purposes of fieldnotes described above, however, do not guide the structure of these layers of the field text to a great extent. Instead, the fieldnotes should, like the interview transcripts, should rely mainly on narrative data—in other words, fieldnotes constitute the story of the researcher's experience of inquiry and serve as a record of the researcher's own construction of meaning. This narrative quality is apparent in the following example of a fieldnote recorded by Steeves during the caregiver study. (Fieldnotes are rough documents in terms of language and grammar: it is more important to get information inscribed in a form that the investigator can read than it is to polish it up for a wider audience.)

June 6—Lewis Visit

The yellow bungalow sits off the road and is invisible if you are not looking for it. It is difficult to write about this visit for me. It was not a family I immediately hit it off with. I did not immediately dislike them but was put off by her [the person dying of cancer] and did not find him [the husband and caregiver] particularly a good informant. I am not sure what it was about him but she was rather domineering. She was a large lady who sat in the middle of the front room and dominated it. She outweighed him by 50 lbs. or more. She was going to sleep in her chair during my talk with him. I hinted that we could talk in the other room and he declined. But she got a phone call and kept talking about going to another room to talk but didn't. So Warren (called Skip by his friends but Warren by his wife who does not like the name Skip) and I started to talk and she complained to the person on the phone that we were too loud and disturbing her. She had to have help getting to the next room. It was a long distance call from her son about car insurance because of a small wreck they had just had ([discussed] on the tape [of the interview]).

She has a small very ugly dog—almost all its hair is gone and it has an ugly growth around its chin—who sits on the furniture and barks at me until she lets it out so it can stand on the front steps and bark. She calls the dog "Momma."

There was the sense that it was her house. A very small house that I really only got to see the front room of. There was little decoration on the walls except pictures of her children (he has none) and a little plaque that said at the top "ordination" but was unreadable [beyond] that. The furniture was far too big for the little room. There were at least four chairs (one a big recliner) and a couch in a very small room. A little half-door divided the kitchen from the front room, a door to keep the dog out of the kitchen. Was the opposite of what I would have expected. When the phone call was over [she] came back into the room and broke into our conversation to correct Warren on details and add a comment about what a good life they had had [together].

At the end of the conversation, Skip walked out with me and over towards his garden. A big well-kept garden by my standards even though he called it small. It was clear he would rather be outside than in with his wife. I am rather sympathetic towards him but I am frustrated because he does not spend time examining his life. No thoughts to the future at all. Perhaps it is too frightening to talk about.

He talked sitting in a chair next to me with his hand over his mouth the entire time. Hard to interpret but surely subconscious—guilt, conspiracy—who knows?

Fieldnotes need to be written as soon as possible after any period of observation. The importance of this statement cannot be overemphasized. One of my students from Taiwan told me, "there is an old saying that the best memory is not as good as the lightest ink." If put off too long, writing fieldnotes becomes more difficult, and the notes become less accurate and complete. It is important to build in time for the writing of fieldnotes during days of data collection. In my experience, 2 to 3 hours of writing fieldnotes for each hour in the field is a good guideline.

A technique that has worked well for me is iterative. In the nursing home study, every hour or so in the field, I would excuse myself from social interaction and find a place, such as an empty room, to jot down words and simple phrases for a few minutes in a small, unobtrusive notepad that fit in my shirt pocket. These brief notes served as reminders and memory triggers. Immediately after leaving the field, I expanded on these notes, fleshing them out, so to speak. Finally, each evening I would sit at my word processor, using the second draft of my notes, and expand even further and describe my experiences, observations, and reflections in greater detail. It was this third iteration of the fieldnotes that became part of the field text for analysis.

In both the caregiving and bereavement studies, Steeves recorded his observations and reflections on audiotape immediately after each interaction with an informant. After the tapes were transcribed, Steeves would elaborate as necessary in greater detail. Cohen also has taped fieldnotes in several of her studies.

Fieldnotes and documents, the latter discussed in the following section, can be analyzed in the same way as interview transcripts. The steps of analysis are detailed in the next chapter. Both fieldnotes and documents are invaluable in writing about the context of the findings, allowing detailed description of the circumstances surrounding the specific lived experiences studied.

For readers interested in more discussion about fieldnotes, Taylor and Bogdan (1984) offer numerous practical tips on recalling observations and recording fieldnotes. A very interesting volume by several sociologists details the processes of writing, coding, and analyzing fieldnotes in a way that is readily accessible to novice researchers (Emerson, Fretz, & Shaw, 1995). For more advanced readers, an edited volume by Sanjek (1990) considers philosophical and practical issues in the construction and use of fieldnotes from an anthropological perspective.

FIELD DOCUMENTS

A final layer of the field text consists of any documents that are collected in the field. I mean documents in the broadest sense—anything that is fixed in some permanent form that can be looked at or viewed again in some way by the researcher. This includes not only writing but also photographs, videotapes, and artwork.

Some documents are obvious. If informants are being recruited from an institution, such as a hospital, hospice, or nursing home, there are brochures and forms that have been seen by informants and that should be collected. Although I have not used medical records in my research, they can be used in some inquiries.

Other documents are serendipitous discoveries that cannot be predicted in advance. In my experience, these documents were given to me by the informant as a result of a phenomenon that Dumont (1978) noted in his own experiences with fieldwork. As Dumont pointed out, while the researcher is going about the work of understanding what is meaningful for the informants, the informants are doing the same regarding the researcher's horizon. In the nursing home study, an informant handed me a letter she had clipped from a newspaper. The letter spoke of the irony of nursing home residents, aware of their own impending deaths, spending their last days being entertained by the staff with trivial games and amusements in the name of recreational therapy, because no one was comfortable talking about death.

In addition, interpretive phenomenologists have pointed out the usefulness of experiential descriptions in literature, including fiction, poetry, and autobiography, to offer insight about the experience that is the phenomenon of concern (van Manen, 1994). There is a growing literature about various aspects of living with illness. Although collecting and cataloging this literature in a comprehensive way is beyond the scope of most hermeneutic phenomenological projects, some of the literature can be incorporated into the field text when it is particularly salient for the informants in the study. When informants mention specific literature that they have read and that has affected their experience, that literature should be collected and studied.

ADVICE FOR NEW RESEARCHERS

Active inquiry in the hermeneutic phenomenological method demands that researchers master several techniques to construct the field text, which serves as the basis of analysis. Interviewing, observing, and collecting field documents were described above, and the importance of narrative data was emphasized.

Technical skills increase through practice. Researchers new to this method should practice interviewing and observing before entering the field. I particularly recommend these exercises:

- Interview a friend or fellow student and record it. Try to elicit stories from the interviewee, focusing on aspects of life that are not usually talked about, such as past loss. Transcribe the interview yourself so that you become familiar with your conversational style. Pay special attention to portions of the interview where you change the subject or abruptly interrupt the narrative flow.

- Go to a public place with a friend or fellow student. Spend a half-hour observing the social activity and the setting. Be together but do not speak about what you observe. Separately, spend an hour or two writing up fieldnotes about your observation. Sit down and compare them, noting the similarities and differences.

- Arrange to have a conversation for a half-hour with a few other people who allow you to tape-record it. Spend an hour or two writing up fieldnotes that describe the conversation and who said what. Listen to the recording and compare with your notes.

The point of each of these exercises is to improve skills of listening, remembering, and writing. Practicing in this way will familiarize a new researcher with the discipline required to construct an adequate field text. Reviewing the results will familiarize a new researcher with the critical attention and reflection about interviews and fieldnotes that are necessary to the whole process of hermeneutic phenomenological inquiry.

7

HOW TO ANALYZE THE DATA

MARLENE Z. COHEN
DAVID L. KAHN
RICHARD H. STEEVES

The process of phenomenological analysis will be discussed and illustrated in this chapter. Process normally implies a beginning and
end, as well as a series of stages or steps by which one can measure progress. In hermeneutic phenomenological analysis, this notion of process
is tricky. There is a beginning of sorts—analysis begins with data collection. As the researcher begins constructing the field text through interviews and observation, the researcher cannot help but begin reading
this text (and hence analyzing and interpreting its meaning). There is an
ending in the narrative text that is produced, although this ending is
understood as tentative and historically bound. The process of analysis
can be characterized as moving between two metaphors—that of a field
text, constructed through the activities of data collection, and that of a
narrative text, which is meant to convey the researcher's present understanding and interpretation of the data to all other readers and which
stands alone as the findings of a hermeneutic phenomenological study.

This process, however, is not linear, although attempts to describe analysis inevitably are.

This chapter opens with a discussion of the overall orientation to interpretation that underlies the hermeneutic phenomenological approach. Second, issues regarding data management are discussed. Next, a style of data reduction and analysis appropriate to the hermeneutic phenomenological method is presented and illustrated with examples from our work. This is presented as an example and not as the only way to conduct analysis, as individualized styles are developed with experience. Finally, the use of teams in hermeneutic phenomenological research and data analysis is considered.

ORIENTATION TO INTERPRETATION

The goal of the analysis is a thick description that accurately captures and communicates the meaning of the lived experience for the informants being studied. A thick description is one that captures the experience from the perspective of the informant in its fullest and richest complexity (Denzin, 1989; Geertz, 1973). The idea of a dialectic process often referred to as the hermeneutic circle underlies hermeneutic thinking and provides guidance for this interpretative effort (Gadamer, 1976; Kockelmans, 1975; Ricoeur, 1981).

The hermeneutic circle is a metaphor that guides the process of inquiry on several levels. Analysis begins as parts of the text are understood in relation to the whole text and vice versa. Then, the individual texts are understood in relation to all the texts and vice versa. The researcher begins with a vague and tentative notion of the meaning of the whole of the data and with the reflexive awareness that this notion is an anticipation of meaning. This awareness causes a dialectical examination of parts of the data to understand better the whole. With a better understanding of the whole, examination of different data or the same parts of the data at a deeper level drives the analysis ahead. This is the hermeneutic circle as it continues throughout analysis (Kockelmans, 1975; Steeves & Kahn, 1995). As Geertz noted (1988), ideally, the hermeneutic circle suggests a continuous dialectic in analysis. He described the process as focusing attention alternatively "between the most local of local detail and the most global [of theoretical] structure in such a way as to bring them into simultaneous view" (p. 69).

In other words, an understanding of the hermeneutic circle requires the investigator to consider the meanings of the smallest units of data in terms of ever-increasing larger units of data and vice versa. For example, in Steeves's study of bereaved people, an African American participant explained that she buried her husband in the backyard where she could "see him from the kitchen window." The statement has meaning standing alone. She had a strong emotional attachment to her deceased husband. But a look at the larger context of that interview changes the interpretation by adding to it. Much of the interview had been about the participant's legal difficulties with her sister about ownership of the land and house in which the participant lived. Burying her husband in the yard was in some sense an act of claiming the land.

The hermeneutic circle metaphor also leads the researcher's analysis outside the context of the individual interview as well as the context of the individual participant. For instance, it was also important to understand that for this woman who buried her husband in the yard, there was no idea of sacred ground. African American Baptist churches did not include that precept in their beliefs. Also, in the last half of the 20th century, burying the dead for African American southerners was problematic. Some families had buried their dead on the family farm, but when good economic conditions in the North began to draw young people away, homes were lost because they were abandoned or were leased or rented to local farmers. Families returning from the North could not find the grave sites, which were now in the middle of wood lots and hay fields. When African American churches were built in the South, they were often built on land donated by White landowners. The land never really belonged to the Black congregation but was on loan. Family members were hesitant to establish church graveyards on land they did not own. Thus, it is in these economic, social, cultural, and theological contexts that the participant's decision to bury her husband in the yard in view of her kitchen window must be understood.

Using the hermeneutic circle as a means of interpreting data means that the smallest statements must be understood in terms of the largest cultural contexts. It also means that all the contexts in between must be taken into consideration; the person, the family, and the community must be considered. Each interview and each fieldnote is read and thought about individually. Then, the whole of the data is read, both to see how the individual fieldnote can be elucidated by an understanding of the whole and to see how the whole can be made more understandable by the individual. This process should be repeated in terms of all that the researcher can learn about the broader culture of the participant from any and all sources.

Some philosophers have argued that the hermeneutic circle is the ontological basis of how humans understand each other in everyday life (Bleicher, 1980; Schwandt, 1994). This is the basis of the metaphor of horizons used by Gadamer (1976) and Merleau-Ponty (1962) in phenomenology. Human beings understand worlds in a way that involves their perception of self as the center of the world present at hand, inseparable, and stretching in all directions (Heidegger, 1962). Humans interpret the horizons of others through a circular, hermeneutic process, using trial and error, questioning and correcting, along with the shared meanings that are available to all members of a culture. Hermeneutic phenomenological researchers use a similar process, but relying on the metaphor of texts introduced previously, they document more rigorously the steps of interpretive understanding as they attempt to incorporate a portion of the participant's horizon of experience into their own.

In other words, data analysis begins with data collection. The tentative understandings of the data that emerge from initial analysis should be subjected to scrutiny as more data are collected. This, in turn, leads to further refinement of these understandings, which will again be scrutinized in light of new data. The tentative understandings should always be in written form. Not only do these writings serve as a record of the analytic process, but also, as van Manen (1994) has described it, the act of writing itself forms the research process in hermeneutic phenomenology.

DATA MANAGEMENT

Hermeneutic phenomenological studies generate a significant amount of qualitative data. In the studies the three of us have conducted, together and separately, we have learned the importance of using an organized system to manage the data. This management involves several principles. First, the interview data and the fieldnotes should be converted into digital form as soon as possible after they are gathered. This allows the data to be copied and stored in multiple places in both digital (computer file) and hard-copy forms. Audiotapes of each interview need to be transcribed verbatim, and the accuracy of the transcription should be thoroughly checked. Printed transcripts should be formatted so that there are wide margins to accommodate writing notes in the margins. It is useful to number the pages and lines, a feature in most formatting aspects of word-processing programs. Identifying speakers with some brief identification is also helpful for quick retrieval. For each study, it is important that the data management system used be developed as soon as possible, preferably before data collection actually begins (see Huberman & Miles, 1994, for a detailed discussion of this point).

In the past two decades, a variety of computer software programs have been developed to assist with data management aspects of qualitative research. Tesch (1990) provided a comprehensive review of this software. Programs have been developed for different types of studies. For example, *NUD*IST* (non-numerical unstructured data indexing, searching, and theorist) (Richards & Richards, 1994) was designed for grounded theory; *Ethnograph* (Seidel & Clark, 1984) was designed for ethnographic studies; and *Martin* (Diekelmann, Schuster, & Lam, 1991) was developed for phenomenological research. But the use of each program has quickly crossed these traditional boundaries. For example, each of us knows phenomenological researchers who have successfully used each of these programs for data management and analysis. In general, these programs assist researchers in adding theme labels to text so that such text is more easily retrieved and grouped during analysis without the need for manual cutting of transcripts and other data. Which program is used is mainly, in our opinion, a matter of preference, availability, and the time needed to learn the specifics of a program. Readers who want more discussion of the use of computers in qualitative research are advised to consult the comprehensive text by Fielding and Lee (1991). We also know other successful phenomenological researchers who get by with database and word-processing software to manage their qualitative data. And at least one of us still prefers physically cutting up the field text and regards forming a mess of actual piles of text excerpts on slips of paper as crucial to the analytic process.

DATA ANALYSIS

Analysis in the hermeneutic phenomenological approach involves moving from the field text, created by data collection, to a narrative text that is meant to stand alone for other readers (Ricoeur, 1981). The movement from one text to the other takes the whole time of the study, reading and rereading the field text in multiple ways and no set order (Steeves & Kahn, 1995). As the multiple readings of the data go on, writing and rewriting of the narrative text occurs. For researchers new to this method, however, an ordering of analytic steps is useful.

Analysis actually begins during interviews, when researchers are actively listening and thinking about the meaning of what is being said. Possible labels for these meanings may begin to be constructed. Informants and others are often asked to validate these labels, as well as labels that result from more careful analysis of transcripts of all interviews.

This more careful analysis continues as the researcher simply reads through data several times or more. This phase is sometimes called "immersing oneself in the data." The aim of this immersion is the establishment of an orienting gestalt or, in other words, some initial interpretation of the data that will drive later coding of the data in subsequent phases of analysis (Barritt et al., 1983, 1984; van Manen, 1984, 1994). In this first phase, the researcher identifies the essential characteristics in the data from each interview or encounter with an informant (Kockelmans, 1975; Steeves, 1992b). It is important to emphasize the importance of this aspect of analysis for all subsequent activities.

Next, there is a phase in analysis that can be called data transformation or data reduction. This step in data analysis involves some decision making on the part of the researcher concerning what is relevant and what is not. The process is similar to editing. Transcriptions of the interviews typically include digressions, abrupt changes in topics, and verbal ticks. The researcher can reorganize the interviews to place together discussions of the same topic, eliminate digressions that are clearly off topic, and simplify the spoken language of the informants (eliminate "you know" for instance) without changing the unique character of it. After these steps, the data can be subjected to the line-by-line coding necessary for thematic analysis with reduced chance of being overly reductionistic and losing sight of the meaning of the whole encounter.

Thematic analysis, the next phase in analysis, is based on the Utrecht school of phenomenology (Barritt et al., 1983, 1984; van Manen, 1984, 1994). Once an understanding of the overall text is obtained, phrases in the text are underlined, and tentative theme names are written in the margin of the text. Data are examined line by line, and all important phrases are labeled with tentative theme names.

This phase of the analysis requires that the investigators label themes and extract passages that have similar themes to be able to look at them together and alongside passages that have the same label but are separated from the rest of the text. The following example illustrates this process. In a recently completed study, Cohen worked with doctoral students to analyze interviews conducted with people who had had bone marrow transplantation. The text excerpt in Figure 7.1 is from the end of the first interview with a 44-year-old Latina health resources director, whom we called Ana. Ana, a married mother, had three young children. She had breast cancer, which was treated first with surgery and then with chemotherapy, radiation, and finally a bone marrow transplant. She was interviewed after transplantation.

The process this example illustrates is that the text of the interviews was analyzed line by line, as shown with Ana's text. Important phrases were underlined (in italics here), theme names were added to the margins, and then passages were cut out of the text. Piles were made of passages with similar labels, and groups of text were sometimes subdivided. An example of this is the terror this woman described. Other informants' language and descriptions were less passionate, and together the passages were labeled as the theme "fears." This came to be seen as fear of death, along with several fears that underlay that fear.

This passage illustrated several themes, three of which have been developed into manuscripts. Cohen and Ley (2000) wrote about the many fears faced by people who have bone marrow transplantation. The overarching fear is fear of death, often related to cancer recurrence. This was illustrated above by the fear of leaving the hospital and not having someone "constantly looking at you to make sure that the cancer isn't back." However, this overarching fear also subsumed other fears, not discussed in this one excerpt. The fear of the unknown, which came from being

 1 Q: Tell me what I've missed. Have there been things that I

 2   haven't asked you about or areas that I haven't covered or things

 3   that you'd like to add?

 4 A: Gosh no. We talked about the nurses and the doctors.

 5   No, I think . . . there is one, maybe two things . . . I kind of wonder

 6   about them sometimes. I don't really know what the deal is.

 7   It's afterwards. *After the bone marrow transplant and the*

 8   *radiation,* it's like for a while *you feel like Dr. Jekyll and*

 9   *Mr. Hyde* because a part of you says I'm so *glad to be finished* with

10   it and *if I never see that place again it will be too soon* type of

11   thing. So part of you feels that way. And then another part of

12   you feels that you have an *umbilical cord to this place* and

13   you're *terrified not to be here,* because as long as you're here

14   *somebody is constantly looking at you to make sure that the*

15   *cancer isn't back.* And so you're terrified I suppose, *like a kid*

16   *whose parents tell him he has to move out of the house.* You're

17   terrified that *how do I know it isn't growing back right this very*

18   *second.* Nobody is looking at it. And so you've got this bizarre

19   feeling that's like one way and the other. And *you catch a cold*

20   *or you have a sore throat and your inclination is that you want to*

21   *pick up the phone and call the doctors* that you had at [the

22   cancer center] then you think well, I don't think I'm supposed

23   to. I think I'm supposed to go to the *regular MD.* But he *just*

24   *seems so vanilla* compared to the people here. He *just seems so*

25   *ordinary,* I guess. So that's kind of a weird thing.

26   I suppose if I was going to talk about *educating the*

FIGURE 7.1. Excerpt From Interview With Line Numbering
to Facilitate Analysis

27   *family and educating the patients, I would go beyond the*

28   *transplant and try to educate them as well on how to bring*

29   *closure.* I don't think anybody does that. I don't think there's

30   anybody that gives you any information or helps you or works

31   with you through closure. Closure appears to be an *individual,*

32   *independent* whatever you do with it, and if you don't do

33   anything with it then I guess you don't have closure. Nobody

34   seems to address it. It's kind of like, after the radiation I

35   continued to attend the *support group meetings* for . . . I started

36   *missing* a lot of them because I was *back at work* and stuff and

37   they were always held on Mondays, and that's always a travel

38   day and that kind of stuff, so I missed more of them than I came

39   to, than the number that I attended. *Then one day I thought*

40   *well, so how long do you go to these things or how long do you*

41   *continue to like call* [the oncology physicians] if you get sick?

42   At what point do you begin to see a regular General Practitioner

43   outside of [the cancer center]? How do you break loose; *when*

44   *do you break loose? Are you supposed to break loose?* How do

45   you go about it? I didn't know . . . one day I was *sitting in the*

46   *support group,* and they were going around the table talking, and I

47   kind of looked around, and I thought, "Of the people that were

48   *the original ten or twelve that started the group, there were three*

49   *including myself, and I thought, "I think it's time to move on."*

50   So when it got to be my turn to talk, I said, "Well, I just *want to*

51   *say goodbye* because I won't be back after today" and that's

52   fine. I don't have any problem with it, *but I sort of just did it on*

53   *the spur of the moment not because there was any guidelines.*

unprepared physically and emotionally, was illustrated again by Ana in the following excerpt:

> That was a big surprise to me that the emotional feelings about the whole experience would be so strong, would last so long. Maybe they're lasting a long time because they never really got released anywhere. . . . You let it out a little tiny bit at a time. I didn't realize that the chemotherapy would be so difficult as it was physically and mentally and emotionally. It was very, very difficult.

Another example from this research was analysis of the following passage from Connie, a 22-year-old student who had a bone marrow transplant. She said,

> I got the shingles. I never knew what shingles were, and I didn't know, and I got so scared. And I come there, and they're like, "Oh, don't worry, that usually happens to bone marrow transplants after." And I said, "see, no one told me this. You should have told me because I started stressing out." . . . I just think they should prepare people before they go in, of what is going to happen to you after, and what really a transplant is.

This passage was identified as an exemplar and coded as "information needs." Exemplars are defined as bits of textual data in the language of the informant that capture essential meanings of themes. This passage was included in the theme that was finally labeled "a range of needs for information." As this example illustrates, analysis of data includes elements or categories within themes. The element "information needs" together with other elements made up the theme "a range of information needs." Many passages were found in these interviews that dealt with patients' needs for information. Analysis made it clear that there were patients who believed staff would tell them what they needed to know and that they need not ask any questions. Another group wanted to know as much as possible. They mobilized resources outside the hospital to obtain the information they wanted. And finally, another group had questions and fears and was not always clear about what to ask, how to ask it, or who might provide the information or reassurance they wanted. Connie's text above showed she was in this group.

In addition to this range of needs for information, other themes emerged in the analysis that related to patients' information needs. (This portion of the analysis was conducted with a doctoral student,

Anita J. Tarzian, and the project was conceived by and conducted with the important assistance of Peggy Iwata, a clinical nurse specialist.) This included the following themes:

1. The need to know and the fear of knowing
2. Everybody's different—a fine balance
3. Someone who has been there
4. The burden of teaching family

Thus, the theme of "patients' information needs" was described as having five components, which can be called subthemes, categories, or elements of the major theme (Tarzian, Iwata, & Cohen, 1999). Informants' descriptions also conveyed the spiritual aspects of the experience of bone marrow transplantation (Cohen, Headley, & Sherwood, 2000). This included questions about the causes and consequences of the disease and reappraisal of life as the meaning and significance of life and death are examined in the context of loving relationships, losses, and hope.

Publications by Riemen (1986) and Barritt et al. (1984) are two excellent examples that illustrate the analysis process. Both articles described the analysis process and illustrated it with examples. Riemen included illustrations in her manuscript, which showed how she went from the text to significant statements to formulating the meaning of caring in her research.

In a large project, it may also be useful to conduct descriptive analysis of demographic data. For example, in our multisite phenomenological study of oncology nurses, we interviewed 38 nurses. Our manuscripts included descriptive statistics about these nurses, such as their age range, education, work setting, job classification, and other demographic features (Cohen, Haberman, & Steeves, 1994).

Finally, the process of writing and rewriting is crucial to interpretive phenomenology (van Manen, 1994). The movement from identification and comparison of themes to a coherent picture of the whole occurs through this reflective process of writing and rewriting. As each investigator gains insight and a tentative understanding of the meaning of the informants' experience, as conveyed through the exemplars and in the themes, the understandings should be summarized in written memos that are circulated among team members. These memos serve to document the hermeneutic process and drive the transformation of the field text to a coherent narrative text (Steeves & Kahn, 1994).

Fieldnotes and relevant narratives (as described in the previous section) are used to contextualize and clarify the themes from the interview data during the process of writing and rewriting. As will be described in Chapter 8 on reducing bias, themes can be verified with the informants to ensure that the themes appropriately capture the meaning that the informant sought to convey. As questions arise in the analysis, the informants should be contacted for clarification when this is possible. When it is not possible for informants to do this verification and clarification, such as when informants are terminally ill, for example, other procedures need to be implemented (see Chapter 8).

TEAMWORK

Some of our work has illustrated how a team of investigators can conduct phenomenological research. In one research project, Cohen worked with a multisite research team. The project began with the entire team meeting and interviewing each other (Cohen et al., 1994). Prior to beginning the interviews, Cohen and other interviewers examined their prejudices about working with patients who have cancer by interviewing each other, using the interview guide with modifications to fit someone who might not be working with patients who have cancer. For example, a question asked of nurses, the informants in this study, was "What is it like for you to work with patients with cancer?" Nurses were asked to describe a particular example of their work with a particular patient. In our interviews, because we were not all working clinically with people with cancer and because our purpose was to practice interviewing skills, we asked, "Describe what you believe it is like for nurses who work with persons who have cancer." All research team members reviewed and discussed the taped interviews. After each interview, strengths, weaknesses, and alternative approaches that could be used in future interviews were also discussed. The goal of this training was to develop interviewers whose styles are equivalent. The interviews were reviewed prior to beginning the study and during the study to ensure that the interviewers had the skills to obtain the data needed from the interviews.

Areas of interviewing that are important to address include reducing interviewer bias, preventing the introduction of assumptions and leading statements, reflecting informants' views rather than suggesting views, and helping informants elaborate and clarify their perceptions. The principal investigator (PI) needs to continue to review audiotapes and discuss them with interviewers throughout the project. This procedure, discussed by Tripp-Reimer (1985) and used by Cohen and Steeves in prior research, has been successful in obtaining rich phenomenological data. Having other interviewers in addition to the PI creates distance between the PI and the data, which is a disadvantage. This approach, however, has the advantage of training doctoral student interviewers, as well as the potential of training nurses to obtain these skills. It is important that the PI do many of the interviews, perhaps following a subgroup of informants intensively, to reduce this distance from the data.

Our work has demonstrated the advantages of having a team work together to analyze a large volume of data. Early meetings are useful and important in establishing working relationships. Data analysis is often best accomplished as a collaborative effort among team members. One person, however, needs to be responsible for coordinating data analysis. This coordination role is necessary given the tremendous amount of textual data phenomenological projects generate. Team members need to work together closely on the analysis. During our breast cancer project, we communicated using e-mail, which allowed transfer of text files from one site to another. As a word of caution, the complexity of this is greater than it may seem. We spent many hours consulting with various computer experts on our campuses to resolve issues of incompatibility among the software programs we were using. The problems were not all solvable. In addition, we had telephone conference calls and one face-to-face meeting over 4 days to complete the analysis and plan future work together. Periodic, perhaps quarterly meetings should be held during a multisite or multimember project. The sites for these meetings should rotate when interviewers and graduate students are involved to allow all of them to participate in the meetings with less travel time and expense. The project should begin with a meeting that includes all interviewers. This will allow team members to conduct the initial training interviews described previously, which help to establish consistent interviewing styles and to expose pre-existing biases.

8

REDUCING BIAS

David L. Kahn

This chapter will introduce the reader to the idea of reducing bias in studies using the hermeneutic phenomenological approach. Given the intended audience for this book, this is an area of discussion I approach with some trepidation. It is an area in which it is too easy for readers (as well as authors) to become lost in literary arguments justifying or disagreeing with the use of particular terminology. There is no agreement among phenomenological or hermeneutic researchers specifically, or qualitative researchers in general, about what to call this whole area or how to discuss it. More precisely, there is no agreement, and indeed there is general disagreement, about the language that should be used in discourse about qualitative research. Whereas I refer to it as reducing bias, other authors refer to it under the rubrics of reliability, validity, accuracy, rigor, goodness, quality, and bias control in qualitative research. Works by Creswell (1998), Lincoln and Guba (1985), and Sandelowski (1986, 1993, 1995), although using different terminology, have been particularly helpful in the development of my own opinions about and practices in reducing bias.

Like other interpretive methods, the hermeneutic phenomenological approach is not grounded in an epistemology that assumes the existence of facts and objective reality in the social world to be like that of the natural world. Part of the horizon in which interpretation takes place includes the researcher's own perspective and the historical context (Koch, 1994). Readers of the narrative text produced by the researcher bring their own perspectives and historical conditions to the act of reading (and interpreting) what the researcher has produced. This is not to say that interpretations in hermeneutic phenomenological research do not aim to be accurate, only that accuracy is contingent and somewhat tentative.

The challenge in producing narrative texts that accurately reflect the dialogue that took place between the researcher and the participants in any given study is to reduce as much as possible the bias the researcher brings to that dialogue. The goal of the hermeneutic phenomenological researcher is to be able to report things as they appear to be as encountered in the field and documented in the field text, rather than as the researcher would have them be.

To move toward this goal involves a constant effort that must permeate all phases of a study. In other words, reducing bias is always on the mind of the researcher, who uses as many techniques and ways as possible, given limitations of time and resources, in the study. These techniques and ways of reducing bias can be separated into two areas for discussion. The first area consists of things the researcher does to identify personal preconceptions, unstated assumptions, and other prejudices that may bias the inquiry. The second area consists of those things a researcher can do to open up the process of inquiry to outside scrutiny. The remainder of this chapter will focus on these two areas in turn.

CRITICAL REFLECTION

The work a researcher does to identify preconceptions, assumptions, and prejudices held has traditionally been called bracketing in the phenomenological literature. In some schools of phenomenology, bracketing is viewed as the first step of inquiry into the phenomenon of interest. All that the researcher assumes and believes about the phenomenon is considered and fixed in written form. This record serves as a checking point as analytic conclusions are made. A rigorous inquiry is one that puts these preconceptions to a test in some way. For example, a researcher can choose participants whose own experience appears to differ from what is expected. Or the researcher can be alert to leading participants in various directions during interviews.

More generally, the process of writing about assumptions and beliefs about the phenomenon beforehand itself causes a process of critical thinking or reflection to begin. This process, really a reflective or critical stance, helps the researcher to become more alert to subtle prejudices. For example, in the initial writing about my own beliefs about heart disease in African American women, before I began that study, I noted that most of my assumptions were based on the image of a middle-class White male much like my own father and grandfather, who suffered from heart disease. I pictured men whose careers had been interrupted by sudden heart attacks, experienced as crushing chest pain radiating down the left arm, along with shortness of breath. And I immediately focused on the biomedical treatments available. Once I understood this about my orientation to the phenomenon, I was able to attend to the different ways the experience of heart disease was described by the participants in my study and the different ways it affected their lives. For example, in my data, there was little talk of pain or pills, and a lot of talk of pressure and spirit.

I also began to notice that these women, to some extent, shared the same image of heart disease I had, that this image was not only a product of personal experience but also a more widely held modern metaphor. It became clear in the analysis that this belief on their part caused them to minimize their own suffering from heart disease, especially in the way they characterized their symptoms.

Another example was a study in which Cohen was the principal investigator (Cohen et al., 1994). The study was designed to understand the meaning oncology nurses found in their work. Prior to interviews of informants, the research team members, who had all practiced as oncology nurses themselves, described their own experiences, using the study interview guide. This discussion was audiotape-recorded, transcribed, and analyzed; this helped ensure that preconceptions "were not introduced to the informants during the interviews or imposed in the data analysis" (Cohen et al., 1994, p. 6).

Thus, the hermeneutic phenomenological method begins, like other phenomenological methods, with bracketing. In the hermeneutic phenomenological method, bracketing is viewed not only as the initial step in inquiry but also as the beginning of a process of ongoing critical reflection. This process is also discussed in literature that focuses on the issue of reflexivity or critical consideration of the influence of the researcher on the products of research (Altheide & Johnson, 1994; Gergen & Gergen, 1991; Lincoln & Guba, 1985; Marcus, 1994).

Continuing the process of reflection is aided by keeping a journal that contains more writing about the same issues that are uncovered during bracketing. This journal is part of the fieldnotes, discussed in a previous chapter, but the extent to which the journal is separated physically (different sections, chapters, notebooks, etc.) and digitally (different files or not) is a matter of researcher preference. What is important is the act of writing about assumptions and prejudices as they are uncovered during the study. Writing forces the researcher to take the time to reflect and critically think about issues of bias reduction during the study.

In addition, the journal also documents the reciprocal influence of the researcher and what is researched (Lamb & Huttlinger, 1989; Marcus & Fischer, 1986). In other words, the journal entries also document changes in the researcher's perspective that occur over the study through dialogue with participants. Once written, the journal entries, as part of the field text, can be read and reread in multiple ways as part of the analytic process.

Here is a guideline, particularly for novices: When considering the reciprocal influence of researcher and what is researched, focus attention on two relationships that are crucial to the qualitative process. These are the relationships of the researcher with participants and with the data (Kahn, 1993). In each journal entry, both relationships can be considered and commented about in writing.

The researcher should pay special attention to issues that are rarely talked about in research reports. Such issues—issues that are taken for granted and go without saying, so to speak—are fertile ground for unexamined bias (Fish, 1979). For example, examination of the relationship of the researcher with the participants, beginning with what Aamodt (1983) and Lipson (1991) called the influence of the researcher on the interview process, should proceed directly to examination of the dialect of the social interactions themselves. For instance, how did elements of gender differences between researcher and participants, social attractiveness, and mutual trust or mistrust enter into the situation? The researcher also should consider the interpretations that participants are inevitably making of the researcher and research project (Dumont, 1978) and how these interpretations affect fieldwork.

Writing about the researcher's relationship with the data needs to begin with recognition of the actual circularity of the hermeneutic process (Kockelmans, 1975). How and when did different understandings emerge, and in how many prior and various forms? In what ways did the investigator challenge his or her own understanding of data, and to what extent were preliminary interpretations tested over the course of the study?

All of the above questions are aimed at developing a reflexive stance on the part of the researcher to the inquiry. A reflexive stance is one that is self-conscious; the researcher is aware of his or her participation in the narratives that are collected and the scientific accounts that are and will be written (Ellis, 1995). This contrasts the normal science stance, which assumes or imagines objective observation to be the point of inquiry and which demands accounts that place the researcher in a third-person position of authority. The products of hermeneutic phenomenological inquiry are instead interpretive accounts created to persuade readers of the validity of the investigator's interpretation (Geertz, 1988).

Ultimately, critical reflection is internal work that the researcher undertakes to make inquiry rigorous. It relies completely on the commitment of the researcher to do whatever works to maintain critical reflection throughout the study and to keep him- or herself fully engaged in the life world of participants. This understanding is reflected in the old and problematic metaphor of qualitative research as "use of the self as instrument" (Kahn, 1993). That this internal work is done is reflected primarily through writing and can be recognized in the writing after the fact. Consider the following fieldnotes I wrote near the end of my fieldwork in the Jewish nursing home study (Kahn, 1990, 1999). In these notes, I considered changes in self related to my relationship with the participants of my study:

> This experience [of fieldwork] has immersed me in ways and understandings of life that were foreign to me. In retrospect, it is painfully obvious that I was guilty as Sally Gadow charged [1983] of beginning this work with a view of the very old as objects somehow apart from my own understanding of human subjectivity, despite my clinical experience with them (or maybe because of my clinical experience). This has changed over the past months as I listened to them talk about their lives. I have given little to them other

than some company and an opportunity to reminisce and pass time. They have given me far more. Through their words, I have glimpsed the essence of my own old age as I carry it now in what and who I care about in this world, and what I will some day lose.

Last week, I heard that Mr. Bassuk died [a pseudonym for a resident with whom I had a close relationship]. And then another informant no longer recognized me or had any energy left to speak. I left the nursing home early. It was a sunny winter day and driving through mid-afternoon traffic had never seemed so good before. It has taken me a week to be able to go back [to the nursing home].

I have noticed that during this study that I have begun reading the obituaries everyday in case someone I know [from the nursing home] is there.

OPENING UP INQUIRY

Opening up inquiry in the hermeneutic phenomenological approach refers to efforts that are made to conform to an understanding of science as a systematic and open human activity. The very word *method*, of course, denotes the understanding that inquiry proceeds methodically or systematically. In the simplest sense, this refers to routine practices, such as verifying transcribed audiotapes for accuracy. The notion of openness means that the system used and the details of methodological and analytical decisions made in any given study can be described explicitly to other scientists. In addition, the hermeneutic phenomenological researcher periodically uses panels of judges, defined as experts on the experience or the method, to check analytic steps, such as the reduction of categories to themes. This is a deliberate and formal opening of the researcher's analysis to others. Opening to others also can be accomplished less formally through the use of colleagues or peers in the scientific community.

The idea that decisions made in a study can be described explicitly is commonly accepted in the literature on qualitative methods. The metaphor most frequently used is that of an audit trail—a metaphor that stresses the need for careful documentation of such decisions during the study (Halpern, 1983; Lincoln & Guba, 1985; Rodgers & Cowles, 1993). In other words, as analysis proceeds, the researcher carefully records these decisions, along with a written justification for making them (Lincoln & Guba, 1985). Lincoln and Guba suggest that another researcher with sophistication in the method but without extensive expertise in the subject area and without personal interest in the study findings be hired to perform an exhaustive audit of these decisions at the end of a study.

For doctoral students and researchers with limited funding, the actual hiring of an auditor may be too costly. However, preparing an audit trail that can be sampled by colleagues or members of a dissertation committee is a useful discipline. An article by Rodgers and Cowles (1993) provides more discussion about the kinds of documentation needed for an audit trail. Besides contextual fieldnotes and the reflective journal discussed previously, Rodgers and Cowles recommend documentation of decisions made about strategies for conducting the study and about the researcher's thought processes in coding and categorizing data.

Panels of judges offer another way to open up the analytic process and identify and reduce investigator bias. Researchers with expertise in qualitative methods or clinicians familiar with the population of the study make good judges. In my own research and my work with Steeves, I have used judges at several points in the movement from more concrete categories to more abstract themes. At each point, the judges were provided with a number of bits of data, ranging from a few lines to a whole narrative, as well as a number of analytic units, categories, or themes, which were carefully defined. The judges were asked to match the data bits with the analytic units. When judges have problems matching, this is a signal to return back to the field text to clarify analysis. I return to the field text (also called an appeal to the original transcript), instead of assuming the judges' position is correct, as judges bring their own biases to the matching effort. For further reading, Hinds, Scandrett-Hibden, and McAulay (1990) have described their effort to ensure "reliability and validity of qualitative research findings" through a process that used judges at four different steps in their analysis.

In some cases, returning to participants to check out interpretations, often called *member checking,* is useful (Lincoln & Guba, 1985). Participants in this technique are judges by virtue of their expertise in the experience. Instead of the matching procedure, description of themes usually can be given to participants for their response. Their responses can often provide more useful data. Disagreements in interpretation should send the researcher back to the field text for clarification, and they should be considered for discussion in reports of the study. Cohen's (1995) discussion of the theme "fear of death" in her study of surgery patients provides an interesting example of such a discussion (p. 170). The patients in Cohen's study were fearful that they might die during or from surgery, but in first interviews, most of them would talk about this fear only in indirect ways. In a second interview, when asked to validate the fear of death theme, the patients opened up and spoke more directly about their fear.

Making use of colleagues can help the hermeneutic phenomenological researcher reduce bias as well. The research process in human science is not solitary. During any study I conduct, there are other members of the research team included because they bring different perspectives. Researchers without the ability to pay team members can still form cooperative alliances with others in the same situation, as doctoral students can team up with other doctoral students. Regular discussions about experiences in the field and ideas about the findings serve to challenge and inform interpretations.

In such discussions, it is important that everyone have access to the field text (after ensuring informant confidentiality, of course). This ensures multiple readers who offer their interpretations as the final narrative is constructed.

As a study progresses and the findings become more coherent, they can and should be communicated to other scholars on a tentative basis through presentations and poster sessions. Questions that arise in these meetings will indicate problems with clarity that, again, return the researcher to the field text.

Ultimately, the findings of an hermeneutic phenomenological study stand alone to be read by others, who begin their own interpretative efforts facing the same problem of meaning, of understanding what the author meant. To the extent that an author has given a thick enough description to readers so that they might understand the interpretation made, that author has also given readers enough access to the field text in the form of original data that the readers may make other interpretations. The question of accuracy transforms at that point into one of utility. It becomes the responsibility of readers of the research findings to decide whether the findings are useful when transferred to their own situations (Lincoln & Guba, 1985). Ultimately, the findings of an hermeneutic phenomenological study can be judged only in the context of the intellectual discourse it joins and creates.

9

WRITING THE RESULTS

RICHARD H. STEEVES

Making sense of data comes with writing about it. Analysis is writing. Logocentric as it may be, this is not such a radical idea. Specifying which ideas are worthy and which are not, arranging the ideas, and making manifest the relationships between ideas is analysis, and it is done through the manipulation of the symbols that constitute those ideas, the words. Only when ideas about data are fixed on paper or disk can the data be analyzed. Because hermeneutic phenomenological researchers are scientists, the form used for the writing of analysis is usually predetermined and rather traditional. But there are some important variations inside this received format. The audience, the form the data take, and the larger goal of the research drive these variations.

SIGNIFICANCE

Most reports on the findings of research begin with a statement of the significance of the study. In simple terms, this is a statement about what the author is doing and why. For research reports, this section is important in establishing the place of the presented study in the canon of research. Researchers and academics in general have a tendency to read papers starting at the back. That is, we want to see the reference list first to see where the writer is located in terms of both method and content. The section of the manuscript titled "Significance" is a literature review that locates the paper in the canon of a particular science and establishes the legitimacy of the writer as a practitioner of the science.

If the audience for the paper is lay or clinical rather than scientific, the significance section takes a different form. Writing a column for the hospice bereavement newsletter about the findings of my studies, I used no references and started with some general statements about the importance of grief, which I hoped my audience would take for granted. When Kahn and I (Kahn & Steeves, 1994) wrote about suffering for the journal *Nursing Outlook,* we did not intend to address a scientific audience, and therefore we spent little time discussing significance in a formal way.

SPECIFIC AIMS

The statement of purpose or the specific aim(s) is a contract. It is a restatement of the contract the researcher used to gain funding or gain the approval of a doctoral committee to do the work. As such, this statement is the measure against which the findings and their interpretations will be judged. For example, did I indeed describe the experiences of men undergoing a bone marrow transplant in a paper reporting the results of a study with that as the aim? This seems an elementary and obvious point, but it is surprising how often this statement of aims is omitted, and the reader has no clear idea what the study was meant to do. Or worse yet, the statement of aims is not congruent with the findings. Researchers sometimes ask one question and return after the analysis with the answer to another. This is not necessarily a bad thing. Discovering in the field that the wrong question was asked and adjusting by asking another question can salvage a study. Often, the new question yields far better and more interesting findings. But this should be a major topic of discussion, and a new set of aims should be articulated. This orienting statement of aims may be put in more or less scientific language, depending on the audience for the paper, but it should be present and prominent for any audience.

METHODS

The methods section of a paper in most scientific journals consists of four basic parts that parallel the proposal: sample, data collection (or procedures), data analysis, and bias reduction. Notice that this is slightly different from the parts expected in a quantitative report. Measurement or instrumentation is omitted, and validity and reliability are collectively referred to as bias reduction.

Rigor is a word used by most scientists to evaluate studies by their peers. What this word means varies considerably from tradition to tradition and perhaps generation to generation, but in general it seems to mean two things. First, do I as a reader know exactly what was done by the researcher? That is, when a researcher states that he or she completed 60 hours of interviews, I want to know where the interviews were conducted. The informant's home is a different kind of place than the researcher's office. Second, do I know why the researcher did what he or she did? Rigor in qualitative research does not mean that all data were collected exactly the same way or analysis was regimented and lockstep. It means that all the decisions made were thoughtful, and alternatives and ramifications were considered. In this case, rigor does not mean stiff or linear but rather well examined or well explained.

Clearly, in nonscientific journals, the rules for reporting research are different. But the usual method of approach is to report findings in a scientific journal first. That way, when presenting findings for an audience of clinicians or an audience of lay people, the researcher can say "for a complete discussion of the methods used please see. . . ." This strategy is used not so much to give readers a source if they want to look up information about the method (something I would guess rarely happens), but rather to testify that the research study has been approved in a blind review by a group of the researcher's peers. Thus, the lay or clinician reader is asked to trust not just this researcher but an anonymous community of scientists.

PRESENTING THE FINDINGS

Numerous variations exist, but generally findings can be presented in two ways. The first could be called the category or theme and quote method. In this method, the overall themes are stated; then, under each theme, the categories, referred to also as elements and subthemes, describing that theme are named and presented. (See Chapter 7 for discussion of themes and categories.) After the first few introductory paragraphs naming the themes and the categories, the paragraphs consist of a topic sentence that restates the category followed by a quote or quotes that illustrate the data used to derive the category. Following the quote, there is often a tie-in statement that explains why the quote is a good illustration of the category, if the relationship is not self-evident. In this way, the categories in each theme are illustrated, and most of the informants are represented in the quotations. See Steeves, Kahn, and Benoliel (1990) for an example of how we have employed this method.

The second method can be referred to as the case study method. Of course, this is not a true case study in that a number of different informants, or cases, contributed to the findings. Occasionally, a single case will be so representative of the major categories and themes that the presentation of that single case can be illustrative of all the categories. The presentation of the data will begin with a long narrative followed by paragraphs naming and illustrating the themes and the categories. These paragraphs will take the same form as the ones above in the category and quotation method, but in the place of the quotations will be brief references back to the single narrative. See Steeves (1996) for an example of how I used a single case study to present the findings of the caregiver study.

Most of the time a single case does not represent all the major categories and themes. Often, three or four case studies are necessary, or in some cases, a fictive narrative that combines the experiences of several informants will be used, and it will be made clear that the narrative is a fiction.

No rule exists for deciding which form the presentation of findings should take. Because the hermeneutic phenomenological method is so closely tied with the idea of narrative, the tendency is to use the case study method. The analysis of narrative, however, is different from the narrative itself, and the findings should be presented in a way that makes them maximally understandable to readers.

Sometimes, it is useful to tell the reader how many informants contributed to each of the categories or even which informants contributed to a certain cluster of categories. This can be a matter of establishing the relative robustness of a category, in the first case, or demonstrating different patterns of experience, in the second case. Both can be useful ways of making the findings more understandable or demonstrating the complexity of an experience. Constructing a grid is a useful and efficient way of presenting these sorts of findings. This technique has been discussed in detail elsewhere (Wise, Plowfield, Kahn, & Steeves, 1992). But the basic process is to let the x-axis represent the informant, identified by a first name or initial, and let the y-axis represent the names of categories as they are grouped in themes. In the resulting grid, the presence of a mark (or perhaps a number if there were multiple contributions to a category from an informant) represents a statement by an informant that contributed to the formation of that category. I am not suggesting that any statistical analysis be done with this sort of data. That would constitute an attempt to understand an experience based on an unreasonable reduction of the data. But the pattern revealed could lead to some interesting conjecture on the nature of the experience.

DISCUSSION

Years ago, a paper I had submitted to a scientific journal was rejected and returned to me with the usual comments from the reviewers. One of the reviewers wrote in criticism that I had "gone beyond my data." I knew what the reviewer meant, and after the natural period of disappointment and ranting that the reviewers had no idea what they were talking about, I decided the reviewer was correct and that I would take it as a compliment. It is the obligation of the researcher to go beyond his or her data, but not in the sense of reaching conclusions unrelated to the data or unjustified by the data. I am using *going beyond the data* to mean thinking what the data might mean in a broader way or using the data as a means of thinking about the broader world. What is the point of doing this kind of work, investigating human experience, if thinking about the human condition in its largest sense is not allowed?

I have come to talk about this kind of thinking as thinking with the data, to borrow a phrase from Geertz (1973), rather than going beyond the data. To do this thinking with the data in the discussion section of a paper, a researcher should place the findings of the study being presented in the context of the findings of other studies. These other studies may be those referred to in the significance section, or they may be other studies that the findings have led the researcher to consider. For instance, a researcher might have set out to explore the experiences of people newly diagnosed with diabetes. The significance section would contain a review of the studies on the experiences of people with diabetes or other chronic diseases. But a major theme in the findings might have been the extent to which these new diabetics were uncertain about their futures. In the discussion section of the paper, a brief review of the uncertainty literature would be in order. Armed with the extant literature on the experience of uncertainty and the contributions made by the new study, the researcher is prepared to think, in writing, with as much of the relevant data as possible, about this human experience.

However, there are two provisos that should be considered when thinking with the data. First, thinking with the data is not the same as making specific recommendations to clinicians or policymakers. Thinking in broad terms with the data about the human condition may be useful for other researchers or theorists or anybody with the intellectual curiosity to care about these issues. But more important, this thinking can change the minds and cultures of clinicians and the public servants who will make specific changes in policy and practice.

Second is the proviso that is best illustrated by the difference between Arthur Conan Doyle and Agatha Christie. The differences between these two mystery writers are numerous, but the one that I am referring to is the amount of information that is given to the reader. Doyle was interested in demonstrating how brilliant Holmes was. Holmes saw things the reader was not aware of and had esoteric information about such things as poisons that was not given to the reader. Christie tells the reader everything that Miss Marple knows. The salient clues are all present. It is for the reader to separate the meaningful clues from the ones that lead nowhere. Agatha Christie should be the model for good research reporting. All the details that are used in the discussion, as the researcher thinks with the data or makes recommendations to theorists and other researchers, should be in the presentation of the findings. The discussion should contain no surprises; all insights must be based on the data presented in the findings section.

REFERENCES

Aamodt, A. (1983). Problems in doing nursing research: Developing criteria for evaluating qualitative research. *Western Journal of Nursing Research, 5,* 398-402.

Altheide, D. L., & Johnson, J. M. (1994). Criteria for assessing interpretive validity in qualitative research. In N. K. Denzin & Y. S. Lincoln (Eds.), *Handbook of qualitative research* (pp. 485-499). Thousand Oaks, CA: Sage.

Barritt, L., Beekman, T., Bleeker, H., & Mulderij, K. (1983). *A handbook for phenomenological research in education.* Ann Arbor: University of Michigan, School of Education.

Barritt, L., Beekman, T., Bleeker, H., & Mulderij, K. (1984). Analyzing phenomenological descriptions. *Phenomenology and Pedagogy, 2*(1), 1-17.

Beecher, H. (1966). Ethics and clinical research. *The New England Journal of Medicine, 274*(24), 1354-1360.

Benner, P. (1984). *From novice to expert: Excellence and power in clinical nursing practice.* Menlo Park, CA: Addison-Wesley.

Benner, P. (Ed.). (1994). *Interpretive phenomenology.* Thousand Oaks, CA: Sage.

Benner, P., & Wrubel, J. (1989). *The primacy of caring: Stress and coping in health and illness.* Reading, MA: Addison-Wesley.

Bleicher, J. (1980). *Contemporary hermeneutics: Hermeneutics as method, philosophy, and critique.* London: Routledge & Kegan Paul.

Brown, L. (Ed.). (1993). *The new shorter Oxford English dictionary.* Oxford, UK: Clarendon Press.

Cohen, M. Z. (1987). A historical overview of the phenomenological movement. *Image, 19*(1), 31-34.

Cohen, M. Z. (1995). The experience of surgery: Phenomenological clinical nursing research. In A. Omery, C. Kasper, & G. Page (Eds.), *In search of nursing science* (pp. 159-174). Thousand Oaks, CA: Sage.

Cohen, M. Z., Craft, M. J., & Titler, M. (1988). Families in critical care settings: Where fear leads to silence. *Phenomenology and Pedagogy, 6*(3), 147-157.

Cohen, M. Z., Haberman, M., & Steeves, R. (1994). The meaning of oncology nursing: A phenomenological investigation. *Oncology Nursing Forum, 21*(8, supplement), 5-8.

Cohen, M. Z., Headley, J., & Sherwood, G. (2000). Spirituality and bone marrow transplantation: When faith is stronger than fear. *International Journal for Human Caring, 4*(2), 41-48.

Cohen, M. Z., Kahn, D., & Steeves, R. H. (1998). Beyond body image: The experience of breast cancer. *Oncology Nursing Forum, 25*(5), 835-841.

Cohen, M. Z., Knafl, K., & Dzurec, L. C. (1993). Grant writing for qualitative research. *Image, 25*(2), 151-156.

Cohen, M. Z., & Ley, C. D. (2000). Bone marrow transplantation: The battle for hope in the face of fear. *Oncology Nursing Forum, 27*(3), 473-480.

Cohen, M. Z., & Omery, A. (1994). Schools of phenomenology: Implications for research. In J. M. Morse (Ed.), *Critical issues in qualitative research* (pp. 136-156). Thousand Oaks, CA: Sage.

Creswell, J. W. (1998). *Qualitative inquiry and research design: Choosing among five traditions.* Thousand Oaks, CA: Sage.

Denzin, N. K. (1989). *Interpretive interactionism.* Newbury Park, CA: Sage.

Diekelmann, N., Allen, D., & Tanner, C. (1989). *The NLN criteria for appraisal of baccalaureate programs: A critical hermeneutic analysis.* New York: The National League for Nursing Press.

Diekelmann, N., Schuster, R., & Lam, S. (1991). *MARTIN user guide, version 2.0.* Madison: University of Wisconsin, School of Nursing.

Dreyfus, H. (1979). *What computers can't do: The limits of artificial intelligence* (rev. ed.). New York: Harper & Row.

Dreyfus, H. L. (1991). *Being-in-the world: A commentary on Heidegger's Being and Time.* Cambridge: MIT Press.

Dumont, J. P. (1978). *The headman and I.* Austin: University of Texas at Austin Press.

Ellis, C. (1995). *Final negotiations: A story of love, loss, and chronic illness.* Philadelphia: Temple University Press.

Emerson, R. M., Fretz, R. I., & Shaw, L. L. (1995). *Writing ethnographic fieldnotes.* Chicago: University of Chicago Press.

Fielding, N. G., & Lee, R. M. (1991). *Using computers in qualitative research.* Newbury Park, CA: Sage.

Fish, S. (1979). Normal circumstances, literal language, direct speech acts, the ordinary, the everyday, the obvious, what goes without saying, and other special cases. In P. Rabinow & W. M. Sullivan (Eds.), *Interpretive social science: A reader* (pp. 243-266). Berkeley: University of California Press.

Fontana, A., & Frey, J. H. (1994). Interviewing: The art of science. In N. K. Denzin & Y. S. Lincoln (Eds.), *Handbook of qualitative research* (pp. 361-376). Thousand Oaks, CA: Sage.

Gadamer, H.-G. (1976). *Philosophical hermeneutics* (D. E. Linge, Ed. & Trans.). Berkeley: University of California Press.

Gadamer, H.-G. (1989). *Truth and method* (2nd rev. ed.) (J. Weinsheimer & D. G. Marshall, Trans.). New York: Crossroads.

Gadow, S. (1983). Frailty and strength: The dialectic of aging. *Gerontologist, 23,* 144-147.

Gallager, S. (1992). *Hermeneutics and education.* Albany: State University of New York Press.

Garfinkel, H. (1972). Remarks on ethnomethodology. In J. J. Gumperz & D. Hymes (Eds.), *Directions in sociolinguistics: The ethnography of communications* (pp. 301-324). New York: Holt, Rinehart & Winston.

Geertz, C. (1973). *The interpretation of culture.* New York: Basic Books.

Geertz, C. (1988). *Works and lives: The anthropologist as author.* Stanford, CA: Stanford University Press.

Gergen, K. J., & Gergen, M. M. (1991). Toward reflexive methodologies. In F. Steier (Ed.), *Research and reflexivity* (pp. 76-95). Newbury Park, CA: Sage.

Gift, A., Creasia, J., & Parker, B. (1991). Utilizing research assistants and maintaining research integrity. *Research in Nursing & Health, 14,* 229-233.

Gumperz, J. J., & Hymes, D. (1972). Introduction. In J. J. Gumperz & D. Hymes (Eds.), *Directions in sociolinguistics: The ethnography of communications* (pp. 1-26). New York: Holt, Rinehart & Winston.

Gurevitch, Z. D. (1990). The dialogic connection and the ethics of dialogue. *British Journal of Sociology, 11,* 181-196.

Halpern, E. S. (1983). *Auditing naturalistic inquiries: The development and application of a model.* Unpublished doctoral dissertation, Indiana University.

Heidegger, M. (1962). *Being and time* (J. Macquarrie & E. Robinson, Trans.). New York: Harper & Row. (Original work published 1926)

Hinds, P. S., & Martin, J. (1988). Hopefulness and the self-sustaining process in adolescents with cancer. *Nursing Research, 37,* 336-340.

Hinds, P. S., Scandrett-Hibden, S., & McAulay, L. S. (1990). Further assessment of a method to estimate reliability and validity of qualitative research findings. *Journal of Advanced Nursing, 15,* 430-435.

Holstein, J. A., & Gubrium, J. F. (1995). *The active interview.* Thousand Oaks, CA: Sage.

Huberman, A. M., & Miles, M. B. (1994). Data management and analysis methods. In N. K. Denzin & Y. S. Lincoln (Eds.), *Handbook of qualitative research* (pp. 428-444). Thousand Oaks, CA: Sage.

Husserl, E. (1970). *The idea of phenomenology.* The Hague: Martinus Nijhoff.

Kahn, D. L. (1990). *Living in a nursing home: Experiences of suffering and meaning in old age.* Unpublished doctoral dissertation, University of Washington, Seattle.

Kahn, D. L. (1993). Technical notes: Ways of discussing validity in qualitative nursing research. *Western Journal of Nursing Research, 15,* 122-126.

Kahn, D. L. (1999). Making the best of it: Adapting to the ambivalence of a nursing home environment. *Qualitative Health Research, 9,* 119-132.

Kahn, D. L., & Steeves, R. H. (1994). Witnesses to suffering: Nursing knowledge, voice, and vision. *Nursing Outlook, 42*(6), 260-264.

Kneipp, S. (1993). *Women who exercise: A phenomenologic inquiry into their adaptation to stress and psychologic strength.* Unpublished master's thesis, University of Michigan, Ann Arbor.

Koch, T. (1994). Establishing rigor in qualitative research: The decision trail. *Journal of Advanced Nursing, 19,* 976-986.

Kockelmans, J. J. (1975). Towards an interpretive or hermeneutic social science. *Graduate Faculty Philosophy Journal: New School of Social Research, 5,* 73-96.

Lamb, G. S., & Huttlinger, K. (1989). Reflexivity in nursing research. *Western Journal of Nursing Research, 11,* 765-772.

Lincoln, Y. S., & Guba, E. G. (1985). *Naturalistic inquiry.* Beverly Hills, CA: Sage.

Lipson, J. G. (1991). The use of self in ethnographic research. In J. M. Morse (Ed.), *Qualitative nursing research: A contemporary dialogue* (2nd ed., pp. 73-89). Newbury Park, CA: Sage.

Mannon, J. M. (1985). *Caring for the burned.* New York: Charles C Thomas.

Marcus, G. E. (1994). What comes (just) after "post"? The case of ethnography. In N. K. Denzin & Y. S. Lincoln (Eds.), *Handbook of qualitative research* (pp. 563-574). Thousand Oaks, CA: Sage.

Marcus, G. E., & Fischer, M. J. (1986). *Anthropology as cultural critique: An experimental moment in the human science.* Chicago: University of Chicago Press.

Mavromataki, M. (1997). *Greek mythology and religion.* Athens: Editions Haitalis.

Merleau-Ponty, M. (1962). *Phenomenology of perception* (C. Smith, Trans.). Boston: Routledge & Kegan Paul. (Original work published 1945)

Mitchell, A. (1997, May 17). Another twist of human rights in the USA. *New York Times,* p. 10.

Morse, J. M. (1991). Qualitative nursing research: A free-for-all? In J. M. Morse (Ed.), *Qualitative nursing research: A contemporary dialogue* (2nd ed., pp. 14-22). Newbury Park, CA: Sage.

Nightingale, F. (1969). *Notes on nursing: What it is and what it is not.* New York: Dover.

Phillips, J. M., & Cohen, M. Z. (1998). *The meaning of breast cancer screening for African American women.* Pittsburgh, PA: Oncology Nursing Foundation, Small Grants Program.

Phillips, J. M., Cohen, M. Z., & Moses, G. (1999). Breast cancer screening and African American women: Fear, fatalism, and silence. *Oncology Nursing Forum, 26*(3), 561-571.

Ray, M. R. (1994). The richness of phenomenology: Philosophic, theoretic, and methodologic concerns. In J. M. Morse (Ed.), *Critical issues in qualitative research methods* (pp. 117-133). Thousand Oaks, CA: Sage.

Richards, T. J., & Richards, L. (1994). Using computers in qualitative research. In N. K. Denzin & Y. S. Lincoln (Eds.), *Handbook of qualitative research* (pp. 516-529). Thousand Oaks, CA: Sage.

Ricoeur, P. (1981). *Hermeneutics and the human sciences* (J. B. Thompson, Trans. & Ed.). New York: Cambridge University Press.

Riemen, D. (1986). The essential structure of a caring interaction. In P. M. Munhall & C. J. Oiler (Eds.), *Nursing research: A qualitative perspective* (pp. 85-105). Norwalk, CT: Appleton-Century-Crofts.

Roche, M. (1973). *Phenomenology, language, and the social sciences.* Boston: Routledge & Kegan Paul.

Rodgers, B. L., & Cowles, K. V. (1993). The qualitative research audit trail: A complex collection of documentation. *Research in Nursing & Health, 16,* 219-226.

Sandelowski, M. (1986). The problem of rigor in qualitative research. *Advances in Nursing Science, 8,* 27-37.

Sandelowski, M. (1993). Rigor or rigor mortis: The problem of rigor in qualitative research revisited. *Advances in Nursing Science, 16*(2), 1-8.

Sandelowski, M. (1995). On the aesthetics of qualitative research. *Image, 27,* 205-209.

Sanjek, R. (1990). *Fieldnotes: The makings of anthropology.* Ithaca, NY: Cornell University Press.

Schutz, A., & Luckmann, T. (1973). *The structures of the life-world.* Evanston, IL: Northwestern University Press.

Schwandt, T. (1994). Constructivist, interpretivist approaches to human inquiry. In N. K. Denzin & Y. S. Lincoln (Eds.), *Handbook of qualitative research* (pp. 118-137). Thousand Oaks, CA: Sage.

Seidel, J. V., & Clark, J. A. (1984). The ethnograph: A computer program for the analysis of qualitative data. *Qualitative Sociology, 7,* 110-125.

SmithBattle, L. (1994). Beyond normalizing: The role of narrative in understanding teenage mothers' transition to mothering. In P. Benner (Ed.), *Interpretive phenomenology: Embodiment, caring, and ethics in health and illness* (pp. 141-166). Thousand Oaks, CA: Sage.

Spiegelberg, H. (1984). *The phenomenological movement: A historical introduction* (3rd ed.). The Hague: Martinus Nijhoff.

Spradley, J. (1979). *The ethnographic interview.* New York: Holt, Rinehart & Winston.

Steeves, R. H. (1992a). Patients who have undergone bone marrow transplantation: Their quest for meaning. *Oncology Nursing Forum, 19*(6), 899-905.

Steeves, R. H. (1992b). Technical notes: A typology of qualitative data. *Western Journal of Nursing Research, 14*(4), 532-536.

Steeves, R. H. (1996). Grief, loss, and bereavement: The Flaharty memorial lecture. *Oncology Nursing Forum, 23*(6), 897-903.

Steeves, R. H., & Kahn, D. L. (1994). Family perspectives: The tasks of bereavement. *Quality of Life—A Nursing Challenge, 3*(3), 48-53.

Steeves, R. H., & Kahn, D. L. (1995). A hermeneutical human science for nursing. In A. Omery, C. E. Kasper, & G. G. Page (Eds.), *In search of nursing science* (pp. 175-193). Thousand Oaks, CA: Sage.

Steeves, R. H., & Kahn, D. H. (1999). Coping with death: Grief and bereavement in elderly persons. In E. A. Swanson & T. Tripp-Reimer (Eds.), *Life transitions in the older adult: Issues for nurses and other health professionals* (pp. 89-109). New York: Springer.

Steeves, R. H., Kahn, D. L., & Benoliel, J. Q. (1990). Nurses' interpretation of the suffering of their patients. *Western Journal of Nursing Research, 12*(6), 714-730.

Steeves, R. H., Kahn, D. L., & Cohen, M. Z. (1996). Technical notes: Asking substantive theory questions of naturalistically derived data. *Western Journal of Nursing Research, 18*(2), 209-212.

Steinbeck, J. (1986). *Travels with Charley: In search of America.* Middlesex, UK: Penguin.

Steinsaltz, A. (1989). *The Talmud, the Steinsaltz edition: A reference guide.* New York: Random House.

Stumpf, C. (1912). *Tonpsychologie.* In B. Rand (Ed.), *Modern classical psychologists.* (pp. 619-623). Boston: Houghton Mifflin. (Original work published 1890)

Suppe, F., & Jacox, A. (1985). Philosophy of science and the development of nursing theory. In H. Werley & J. Fitzpatrick (Eds.), *Annual review of nursing research* (Vol. 3, pp. 241-267). New York: Springer.

Tarzian, A. J., Iwata, P. A., & Cohen, M. Z. (1999). Autologous bone marrow transplantation: The patient's perspective of information needs. *Cancer Nursing, 22*(2), 103-110.

Taylor, S. J., & Bogdan, R. (1984). *Introduction to qualitative research methods: The search for meanings.* New York: John Wiley.

Tesch, R. (1990). *Qualitative research: Analysis types and software tools.* Bristol, PA: Falmer.

Tripp-Reimer, T. (1985). Research in cultural diversity: Reliability issues in cross-cultural research. *Western Journal of Nursing Research, 7*(3), 391-392.

Tripp-Reimer, T., & Cohen, M. Z. (1991). Funding strategies for qualitative research. In J. M. Morse (Ed.), *Qualitative nursing research: A contemporary dialogue* (2nd ed., pp. 243-256). Newbury Park, CA: Sage.

van Manen, M. (1984). *"Doing" phenomenological research and writing: An introduction.* Alberta, Canada: Department of Secondary Education.

van Manen, M. (1994). *Researching lived experience: Human science for an action sensitive pedagogy.* Michigan: Althouse.

Wineman, N., & Durand, E. (1992). Incentives and rewards for subjects in nursing research. *Western Journal of Nursing Research, 14*(4), 526-531.

Wise, C., Plowfield, L. A., Kahn, D. L., & Steeves, R. H. (1992). Technical notes: Using a grid for interpreting and presenting qualitative data. *Western Journal of Nursing Research, 14*(6), 796-800.

Yang, L. (1999). *The lived experience of marital relationship among infertile women in northern Taiwan: A phenomenological study.* Unpublished doctoral dissertation, University of Texas at Austin.

Yow, V. R. (1994). *Recording oral history: A practical guide for social scientists.* Thousand Oaks, CA: Sage.

AUTHOR INDEX

SUBJECT INDEX

ABOUT THE AUTHORS

Marlene Z. Cohen, RN, PhD, is the John S. Dunn, Sr., Distinguished Professor in Oncology Nursing at The University of Texas, Houston, Health Science Center, School of Nursing, with a joint appointment at The University of Texas M. D. Anderson Cancer Center as Coordinator of Applied Nursing Research. She received her PhD in clinical nursing research from the University of Michigan, where she began her program of research on the emotional response to physical illness. Her work has focused principally on oncology since 1990. Using primarily phenomenological techniques in her research, she has conducted several funded studies that examined the meaning of illness from patients' perspectives, described nurses' experiences of working with people with cancer, and compared the perceptions of patients, health care providers, and family members. She is continuing this research aimed at obtaining an accurate understanding of the experience of having cancer and cancer treatment to develop more effective interventions to provide care for patients and their loved ones. In addition, she works with a number of faculty and staff at the Anderson Center on a variety of projects, including the treatment of pain; symptom management, which includes obtaining an understanding of the meaning of symptom management interventions; the use of dream analysis by nurses; improving care for neuro-oncology patients; factors associated with development of prolonged postoperative ileus; and psychological interventions to support patients having bone marrow aspiration.

DAVID L. KAHN, PhD, RN, is Associate Professor and Luci Baines Johnson Fellow at the University of Texas at Austin School of Nursing. He received his PhD in nursing science from the University of Washington in 1990. His dissertation was a study of the experiences of suffering and meaning among residents of a nursing home for Jewish elderly. Subsequent research includes studies of loss and illness in African American elders and women. His current research is a study of cancer patients in a hospice program. He teaches doctoral courses in qualitative research methods and culture and health.

RICHARD H. STEEVES, RN, PhD, is Associate Professor in the Family Division of the School of Nursing at the University of Virginia. He received his PhD from the University of Washington in 1988, where his dissertation was a study of the experiences of bone marrow transplantation patients. His major interest is suffering and how people find meaning in the face of suffering. The complexity and emotional weight of this topic convinced him that hermeneutic phenomenology would provide the best methods for exploring them. This concern with suffering has led to an interest in oncology from the points of view of the patients and the families that care for them. Hospice research has also been an interest because of the suffering and challenge to meaning that the end of life presents. The study of bereavement was a natural extension of that work. Presently, he is piloting an intervention to help recently bereaved people reestablish a sense of ongoing meaning in their lives. His plan is to use hermeneutic phenomenological method in part as a means of evaluating the intervention.